Differential Diagnosis in Abdominal Ultrasound

Differential Diagnosis in Abdominal Ultrasound

R.A.L. Bisset
MB, BS, FRCR

Consultant Radiologist at the North Manchester
General Hospital, Booth Hall Children's Hospital
and Monsall Hospital, Manchester, UK.

A.N. Khan
MRCS, MRCP, DMRD, FRCR

Consultant Radiologist at the North Manchester
General Hospital and Lecturer (part-time) in
Diagnostic Radiology at the Medical School,
Manchester University, Manchester, UK.

Baillière Tindall
London   Philadelphia   Toronto   Sydney   Tokyo

Baillière Tindall
W. B. Saunders

24–28 Oval Road
London NW1 7DX, England

The Curtis Center
Independence Square West
Philadelphia, PA 19106–3399, USA

55 Horner Avenue
Toronto, Ontario M8Z 4X6, Canada

Harcourt Brace Jovanovich Group
(Australia) Pty Ltd
30–52 Smidmore Street
Marrickville, NSW 2204, Australia

Harcourt Brace Jovanovich Japan Inc.
Ichibancho Central Building,
22–1 Ichibancho
Chiyoda-ku, Tokyo 102, Japan

British Library Cataloguing in Publication Data

Is available

ISBN 0-7020-1483-4

Typeset by Photo·graphics, Honiton, Devon
Printed in Great Britain by Richard Clay Ltd
Bungay, Suffolk.

Preface

In the spring of 1986 we undertook a retrospective
review of 45 patients with apparent complex cystic
hepatic mass lesions. Whilst conducting this review we
became increasingly aware of the lack of specificity of
many sonographic findings. When these features were
considered in conjunction with the full clinical history,
physical examination and results of other investigations,
an accurate diagnosis was reached in a high percentage
of cases. The lack of specificity makes the 'gamut'
approach to differential diagnosis very valuable. Since
this time, we have collected 'gamuts' of differential
diagnoses from the literature. Using these differential
diagnoses in conjunction with all the other clinical
information available, we have been able to make an
accurate diagnosis or guide further investigation in
the majority of cases examined. These differential
diagnoses have been valuable in our clinical work and
form the basis of this book.

R.A.L. Bisset
A.N. Khan

We wish to thank our wives and children
  Alison, Alexandra and Charlotte,
  Nazir, Sumaira and Suhail,
for their patience and understanding during our
work on this book.

This book is dedicated to the memory of John
Wolstencroft (1957–1989)

Contents

List of Gamuts

Chapter 3

Chapter 4

Chapter 5

Chapter 6

Chapter 7

Chapter 1

Introduction

Ultrasonography is a uniquely safe and non-invasive means of imaging internal anatomy. Changes depicted include change in organ size, shape, echogenicity and echopattern. This limited number of parameters may be affected by a wide range of disease processes and thus it is not surprising that many sonographic features are very non-specific. In addition, the ultrasonographer must not only demonstrate as many sonographic abnormalities as possible but must also interpret these abnormalities in the light of any clinical information given and the results of other investigations. It is thus not surprising that the diagnostic accuracy of ultrasonography is very observer-dependent and depends not only upon a knowledge of ultrasonography but also of anatomy, pathology, medicine, surgery and allied subjects. Despite the difficulties in reaching a diagnosis the experienced sonographer can frequently considerably shorten the differential diagnosis on clinical grounds making a firm diagnosis or directing the clinician to further relevant investigations. Reasons for errors in sonographic diagnosis include:

The ultrasound scanner is unable to resolve the pathological changes. The scanner may be inadequate for the task e.g. by the use of an inappropriate probe frequency, or the disease process may cause microscopic pathological changes which do not cause an appreciable alteration in echopattern.

Incorrect gain settings or image processing may make normal tissue appear pathological or may mask disease.

Inadequate patient preparation.

Poor examination technique.

Failure to recognize visible sonographic abnormalities.

Faulty interpretation of sonographic findings.

Provided the ultrasound scanner is capable of the required task the majority of variables affecting diagnostic accuracy are under the control of the ultrasonographer.

1.1 SONOGRAPHIC DIAGNOSIS

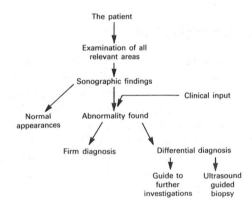

1.1.1 Artefacts

In order to achieve a high degree of diagnostic accuracy the ultrasonographer must be aware of the many artefacts which may be encountered during scanning. These occur due to the physical properties of the

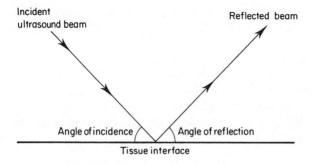

Fig. 1. Specular reflection.

ultrasound beam, technical aspects of scanner construction and assumptions made during image processing which are not always correct.

1.1.2 The origin of artefacts

Ultrasound waves are very high frequency sound waves generated in the ultrasound probe or transducer by the piezo-electric effect. The ultrasound image is derived from the echoes received when an ultrasound beam passes into the body. Each ultrasound pulse is very short and usually lasts less than 1 μs. The transducer then acts as a receiver detecting the echoes of the pulse of sound which it originally emitted. These echoes may arise in several ways:

1.1.3 Specular reflection

When an ultrasound beam encounters a tissue interface it may be reflected in a manner analogous to light hitting a mirror. This is termed specular reflection. The angle of incidence of the ultrasound beam is equal to the angle of reflection (Fig. 1). The reflected beam is only returned to the ultrasound probe when the incident beam is at or near 90° to the tissue interface. The intensity of the reflected ultrasound echoes also depends upon the angle of incidence. Thus when specular echoes are seen they are usually of high amplitude.

For specular reflection to occur there must be an interface between tissues of different acoustic impedence. For soft tissues the acoustic impedance is largely dependent upon the amount of collagen and connective tissue stroma within the tissue. The greatest differences in acoustic impedance occur at air/tissue and tissue/bone interfaces. Reflection of sound is so great at these interfaces that the ultrasound beam is effectively blocked.

1.1.4 Backscatter echoes

Backscatter echoes occur when the size of the reflector is of the same order of magnitude as the ultrasound beam wavelength. The echoes are of low amplitude but return to the transducer with little regard for the angle of incidence of the ultrasound beam.

1.1.5 Rayleigh scattering

Rayleigh scattering is the process of ultrasound beam scattering which occurs when the particles or tissue interfaces causing the scattering are very small in relation to the wavelength of the ultrasound beam (e.g. red blood cells, diameter 6.3–7.9 μm $\times$ thickness 1.9 μm). The intensity of the scattered beam is dependent upon the fourth power of the ultrasound beam frequency and is thus greater at high beam frequencies. It is Rayleigh scattering which is used for Doppler flow

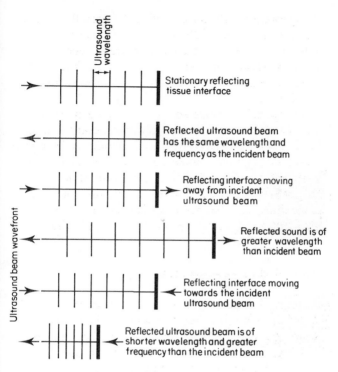

Fig. 2. The Doppler principle.

studies. The Doppler theory is by no means new, it was first put forward by Christian Johann Doppler in 1842. The principle involves frequency and wavelength changes which occur when a waveform, in this case sound, is reflected by a moving target or tissue interface. As Fig. 2 shows ultrasound waves reflected by a moving target will show altered frequency and wavelength depending upon the direction of movement of the reflector relative to the incident beam and the differ-

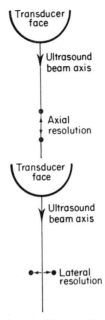

Fig. 3. Resolution.

ence in their velocities. The 'Doppler shift' in frequencies may be used to measure the relative rates of blood flow through vessels. To ensure the optimum signal quality a high frequency ultrasound probe should be used and the sonographer should ensure that the axis of the incident ultrasound beam is as close as possible to the axis of blood flow being analysed.

1.1.6 Ultrasound scanner resolution

The resolution of a scanner is its ability to resolve adjacent structures as separate (Fig. 3). The greater the resolution the closer and smaller the objects which may be differentiated. Resolution is not a constant phenomenon but depends upon the position of the objects in relation to the ultrasound beam and their distance from the transducer. It also differs in the axial and lateral planes.

1.1.7 Axial resolution

The axial resolution is the system resolution measured along the ultrasound beam axis, i.e. perpendicular to the probe face. It depends upon the brevity of the ultrasound pulse and ultrasound beam wavelength. Increasing the ultrasound beam frequency reduces its wavelength and thus improves resolution. Unfortunately increasing beam frequency also causes increased beam attenuation and thus decreased beam penetration. Thus increased resolution is achieved at the expense of decreased depth of view.

1.1.8 Lateral resolution

The lateral resolution of the system is a measure of the resolution of objects or echoes on a plane parallel to the transducer face, i.e. perpendicular to the axis of the ultrasound beam. The lateral resolution depends upon the ultrasound beam width, the size of the transducer face relative to the ultrasound wavelength and the distance from the transducer face. Lateral resolution decreases as the distance from the transducer face increases due to beam divergence. Beam divergence may give rise to artefacts as strong echoes arising outside the main ultrasound beam may be wrongly assumed to have arisen within the beam. Large transducer faces produce less divergent ultrasound beams. Alternatively the beam may be focused electronically.

1.1.9 Incorrect assumptions in image processing:

The speed of sound is assumed to be 1540 m s^{-1} but is in fact variable depending upon the nature of the tissue through which it is passing.

Sound is assumed to travel in a straight line but may be refracted.

All echoes detected by the scanner are assumed to have arisen on the main ultrasound beam axis but they may have arisen in adjacent tissues due to beam divergence.

Artefacts seen in everyday scanning may include:

Acoustic enhancement/shadowing
Reverberation
Electronic noise
Partial volume/beam width artefact
Mirror artefact
Side lobe artefact
Velocity artefact
Refraction artefact
Echogenic focal zone artefact
Paralysis
Comet tail artefact

1.1.10 Acoustic enhancement

The 'swept gain' amplification system used in ultrasound scanners is designed to provide an image of even brightness when scanning homogenous tissue. To this background amplification the sonographer makes adjustments which take into account the nature of the tissues in the section under examination. Frequently different tissues will be present at the same depth in different areas of the ultrasound field. These tissues may attenuate the ultrasound beam differently and thus the intensity of the beam reaching the distal tissues may vary. This is most prominent when the beam passes through a fluid-filled structure such as the gallbladder. The fluid within the gallbladder causes very little attenuation of the ultrasound beam compared to adjacent soft tissues. The beam which has passed through the gallbladder is thus of greater intensity than the beam which has passed through an equal thickness of soft tissues which cause greater beam attenuation. The greater beam intensity distal to the fluid-filled structure gives rise to stronger echoes in the distal tissues and thus echoes arising distal to a fluid-filled structure may appear brighter or 'enhanced' compared to adjacent echoes at the same depth (Fig. 4). Though acoustic enhancement is usually seen behind fluid-filled structures it has been seen to a lesser extent distal to very uniform soft tissues.

1.1.11 Acoustic shadowing

Tissue interfaces which are very good ultrasound reflectors may completely obstruct the passage of the ultrasound beam. As the beam does not penetrate the tissues distal to this interface a shadow results. The reflecting interface is usually seen as a strongly echogenic band with an anechoic area running distally behind it. To cause shadowing the tissue interface concerned must be of a similar size or larger than the width of the ultrasound beam. If a strong reflector is much smaller than the ultrasound beam width then sound waves may pass around it and echoes may then be detected from the distal tissues (Fig. 5). Gas,

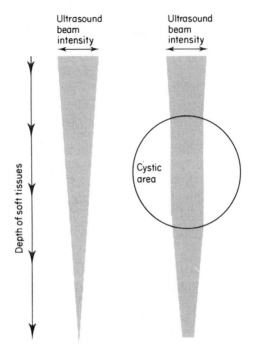

Fig. 4. Distal acoustic enhancement. The ultrasound beam is attenuated as it passes through the body. When passing through fluid the ultrasound beam is subject to little if any attenuation. The beam is therefore stronger distal to a fluid-filled structure than distal to an equal thickness of solid tissue.

bones and calculi are the commonest cause of acoustic shadowing seen in everyday practice. It should be remembered however that small calculi may be seen as echogenic foci without shadowing and the lack of shadowing does not exclude the diagnosis of a small calculus. As the ultrasound beam width is narrowest

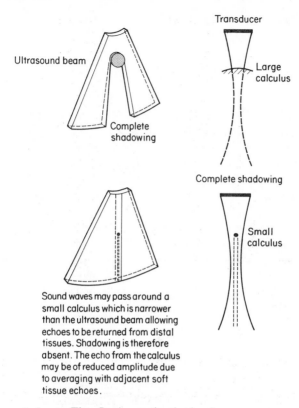

Fig. 5. Acoustic shadowing.

in the focal zone of the beam it is important that any area of interest is kept within this zone. This will increase the chance of seeing shadowing distal to small calculi and also ensure that the area is viewed with the greatest possible scanner resolution.

1.1.12   Reverberation

The transducer face, skin and coupling medium form
acoustic interfaces. Sound passing from the transducer
into the body and echoes returning to the probe from
within the body may be reflected by these interfaces
allowing the sound waves to be reflected back and
forth. These 'reverberating' sound waves may act as
new ultrasound pulses. The majority of echoes generated by the reverberating sound waves are too weak
to be detected by the scanner. At times the echoes are
strong enough to be detected and then artefactual
reverberation echoes will be seen. These are seen as
regular band echoes usually in the near field at 90° to
the beam axis. They are usually multiple with regular
spacing reflecting the distance between the reverberating tissue interfaces. They may occur distal to any
strongly reflecting surface for example the anterior wall
of the fluid-filled bladder.

1.1.13   Electronic noise

An ultrasound scanner, as with any other complex
electronic apparatus, may suffer electronic interference
from adjacent machinery. The artefacts produced by
electronic noise are usually easily recognized, consisting
of radiating lines and echogenic streaks forming patterns which are usually situated on the ultrasound beam
axis. This may be a particular problem if the scanner
is sited adjacent to an operating theatre where dia-
thermy is in regular use.

1.1.14 Partial volume/beam width artefact

The ultrasound beam is of finite width. This may give rise to problems when an object under examination and adjacent tissues both lie within the same part of the ultrasound beam. Echoes arising from the object and adjacent tissues will be presented in the same part of the ultrasound image. This may cause problems particularly when a cyst and soft tissues lie in the same part of the ultrasound beam. Echoes arising from within the soft tissues may give the appearance of debris within the cyst or it may even appear solid and thus be missed (Fig. 6). Small cysts narrower than the ultrasound beam usually cannot be differentiated from solid tissue. Similarly very small echogenic foci within a fluid collection e.g. microbubbles of gas within an abscess, may cause the fluid collection to appear solid owing to summation of the echoes from that volume of tissue.

In order to reduce the risk of misdiagnosis it is essential that all organs are examined in at least two planes preferably at right angles. In addition, changing the patient's position changes the position of abdominal organs in relation to each other. This can be a valuable method of diagnosis when the sonographic appearances raise the possibility of the partial volume effect.

Just as the partial volume effect may give rise to misleading tissue echopatterns the curved contours of adjacent organs may give rise to misleading appearances. The duodenal cap for example may bulge into the gallbladder. If the gallbladder is only examined in a single plane the resulting appearance (Fig. 7) may be mistaken for a gallstone. To ensure that errors such as this do not occur, all areas should be examined in

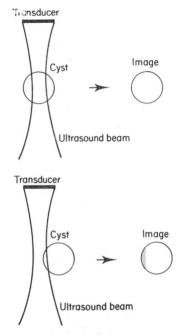

Fig. 6. Partial volume/margin artefact. Scanning both solid tissue and the edge of the cyst simultaneously may give an artefactual appearance of debris within the cyst or a solid appearance.

multiple sections with the patient lying in different positions.

1.1.15 Mirror image artefact

Mirror image artefacts arise when an image arises close to a curved and strongly reflecting tissue interface, for example the diaphragm. The ultrasound beam may

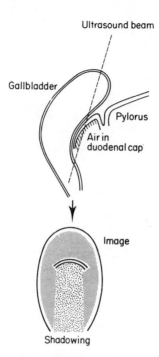

Fig. 7. The ultrasound image is a two-dimensional representation of three-dimensional internal anatomy. Failure to examine the patient in multiple sections may lead to misdiagnosis. Each organ should be examined in at least two planes preferably at 90° as performed with conventional radiography.

then take two paths to reach an object in the field of view (Fig. 8). The second path to the object via the curved reflecting surface is longer than the direct path and gives rise to a second image which lies distal to the curved reflector which caused the artefact.

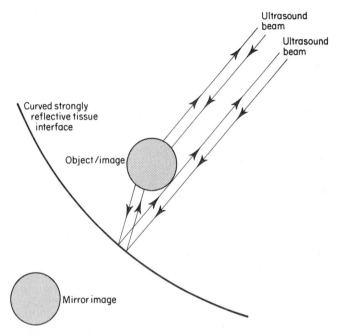

Fig. 8. Mirror artefact. The false image is seen beyond the curved specular reflector due to the second pathway taken by the ultrasound beam.

1.1.16 Side lobe artefact

The ultrasound beam is not uniform but narrows after leaving the transducer to become narrowest in the focal zone. It then widens as it passes deeper into the body. Though the beam may be electronically or mechanically focused some sound waves diverge from the main beam. These sound waves diverging from the main beam are known as the side lobes. They are less intense than the main beam but occasionally strong reflectors within the side lobes may give rise to echoes which may be detected by the transducer. The ultrasound scanner will assume that these echoes arose within the axis of the main beam and will project them as artefactual echoes on the final image. Narrower focused beams are less prone to side lobe artefacts of the partial volume effect.

1.1.17 Velocity artefact

During image processing the ultrasound scanner assumes a constant velocity of sound within the tissues of 1540 m s^{-1}. This assumption is necessary to allow the calculation of distance from the time taken for an echo to return to the transducer. Unfortunately the speed of sound is variable and depends upon the nature of the transmitting medium. The velocity of sound in fat for example is only 1460 m s^{-1}. The variation in the velocity of sound will give rise to distortion of the final image compared to the true internal anatomy and may cause errors of 5 % or greater in the measurement of distances.

1.1.18 Refraction artefact

The ultrasound beam may be refracted in a manner similar to the refraction of light by a prism. The axis of the ultrasound beam is thus not always straight but may cut corners (Fig. 9). This may lead to errors in the registration of the position of origin of ultrasound echoes on the image. Refraction of the ultrasound beam may also lead to beam splitting. This results in an area totally devoid of the ultrasound signal and thus an area of shadowing results on the final image.

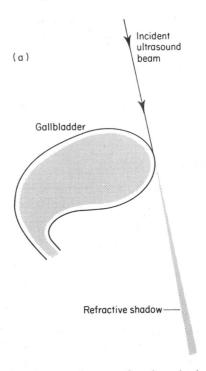

Fig. 9. Refraction artefact – refraction shadow.
(a) A combination of reflection and refraction cause beam splitting giving rise to a 'refraction shadow' due to an area devoid of ultrasound signal.

Refraction and refractive shadowing occur most frequently when the beam strikes the margin of a solid or cystic structure tangentially. This is seen particularly frequently at the gallbladder margin. The presence of refractive shadowing is highly dependent upon the angle of incidence of the ultrasonic beam and thus

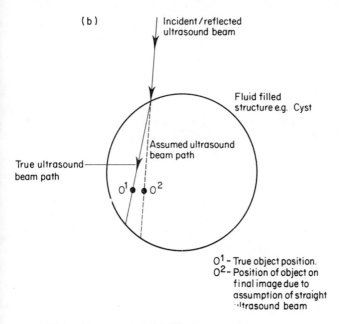

Fig. 9(b). Cysts and fluid-filled structures may act as lenses refracting the ultrasound beam leading to mis-registration of the position of origin of echoes. This effect may occur to a lesser extent with solid structures.

refraction and refractive shadowing are not constant if multiple sections are taken.

1.1.19 Echogenic focal zone artefact

As the ultrasound beam is narrowest in the focal zone the relative intensity of sound per unit area is greater here than elsewhere in the beam. Echoes arising from this area may therefore be of greater intensity than echoes arising from similar tissue interfaces elsewhere in the ultrasound beam.

1.1.20 Paralysis

To generate the ultrasound signal an electrical potential of several hundred volts is applied to the transducer elements. The echoes detected by the transducer are far weaker than the original signal and generate potentials from a few millionths of a volt up to 1 V. These signals are amplified and processed to produce the final image. The amplifier can be overloaded by the high potential used to generate the ultrasound signal and may be temporarily paralysed. This is seen as a block echo in the near field as paralysis occurs immediately after the ultrasound pulse. Paralysis is seen infrequently with modern scanners owing to advanced amplifier design but when encountered it may be overcome by the use of a spacing substance to increase the distance between the transducer and the area of interest.

1.1.21 Comet tail artefact

The comet tail artefact is a form of intense reverberation which occurs between two adjacent surfaces for example the sides of a surgical clip or a small stone. The resultant reverberation echoes are so close to each other that they tend to merge and give rise to a bright 'comet tail' echo extending distally into the ultrasound field behind the structure causing the reverberation.

1.1.22 Comment

To ensure the greatest possible accuracy the ultrasonographer must:

Be fully conversant with the operation of the ultrasound scanner in use, its controls and probes.

Pay constant attention to gain and processing controls during the examination.

Technique should be careful and thorough including changing the patient's position during the examination.

Be fully aware of the physical artefacts and diagnostic pitfalls which may occur.

Discussing the operation of the scanner with the medical physicist in charge of its maintenance is invaluable. The examination of a phantom may also be rewarding.

Chapter 2

Liver, Biliary System, Spleen and Pancreas

2.1 THE LIVER

The liver begins to form early in the fourth week of foetal life. By the ninth week it fills most of the abdomen and accounts for 10 % of foetal weight. At term it accounts for 5 % of the total weight and in the adult this has fallen to 2.5 %. Despite this the liver is the largest single organ in the body weighing 1.5 kg in the adult. Anatomically it is divided into larger right and smaller left lobes separated by the interlobar fissure. In addition there are two smaller lobes. The caudate lobe lies between the inferior vena cava and interlobar fissure posteriorly and the quadrate lobe lies between the interlobar fissure and gallbladder caudal to the porta hepatis. Physiologically the liver is divided by a line from the inferior vena cava to the superior surface of the liver just to the right of the falciform ligament. This divides the liver by portal venous supply into two roughly equal lobes. By this division the quadrate lobe is part of the physiologic left lobe and the caudate lobe lies between the right and left lobes.

The liver is surrounded by peritoneum which is reflected onto the diaphragm and anterior abdominal wall as four ligaments or folds. The falciform ligament passes from the anterior surface of liver to the diaphragm and anterior abdominal wall above the umbilicus. Inferiorly it is continuous with the ligamentum teres. It frequently contains fat and may appear strikingly echogenic. The coronary and right and left triangular ligaments are seen less frequently than the falciform ligament. The liver has a fibrous capsule which is invaginated at the porta hepatis by the portal vein, common hepatic duct and hepatic artery or their branches. The portal vein divides at the porta into right and left main branches. The right lobar vein divides into anterior and posterior branches while the left lobar vein divides into medial and lateral branches. The branching portal veins may be identified within the liver as anechoic tubes with echogenic walls. The bile ducts running with the portal vein branches within the liver are usually too small to be seen except at the porta hepatis unless they are pathologically dilated. Hepatic artery branches also run with the portal venous radicles. They may be identified in the porta hepatis but are too small to be seen within the liver parenchyma. Hepatic veins run directly back through the liver parenchyma to the inferior vena cava. They are seen as anechoic tubes without identifiable walls separate from the portal vein branches though uncommonly they have visible walls.

The normal liver has a homogenous echopattern of relatively fine echoes being slightly more echogenic than renal parenchyma but less echogenic than normal pancreas. The branching pattern of hepatic and portal vein radicles is seen superimposed on this background.

2.1.1 Hepatitis

Inflammation of the liver or hepatitis may take a large number of forms with a wide range of aetiologies.

Clinically hepatitis is usually subdivided into acute and chronic forms.

A   *Aetiology*
ACUTE –

Infective. e.g. Viral, bacterial, parasitic or secondary to the toxic effects of infection elsewhere.

Toxic. Alcohol, chemicals, toxins, drugs and their metabolites.

CHRONIC –

Granulomatous. Primary and secondary biliary cirrhosis. Tuberculosis, histoplasmosis, sarcoid.

Non-granulomatous. Drug reactions, persistent active hepatitis, often viral.

B   *Sonographic appearances*
The liver may appear normal particularly in acute or relatively mild cases. More severe cases show reduced parenchymal echogenicity though less commonly increased echogenicity has been reported. Reduced echogenicity results in a dark liver in which the walls of portal venous radicles appear more prominent than normal giving the 'starry sky' appearance. Hepatomegaly may also occur in severe cases. Uncommonly acute hepatitis may give rise to areas of focal echogenicity which may be mistaken for masses, particularly in cytomegalovirus (CMV) infection and alpha 1 antitrypsin deficiency.

The liver may appear normal in chronic hepatitis. Though cases of reduced parenchymal echogenicity have been recorded in chronic hepatitis increased echogenicity occurs more frequently. In addition to generalized increased echogenicity areas of necrosis give rise to hypoechoic or anechoic foci and these features combined with regenerating nodules may give a generally heterogenous appearance. The general pattern of parenchymal changes may thus vary depending upon the stage of the disease process, particularly as a case of acute hepatitis may evolve into a more chronic form.

2.1.2 The fatty liver

The accumulation of fat in the liver is a non-specific response to a wide variety of aetiologies. This diagnosis can be made histologically when the liver contains more than 7 % fat as lipid vacuoles appear in the cell cytoplasm.

A Aetiology

Toxic – Alcohol, halothane, steroids, tetracycline, chlorinated hydrocarbons.

Nutritional – Obesity, starvation, intravenous feeding.

Metabolic – Diabetes, glycogen storage disease, galactosaemia, lipid storage disease.

Others – Acute fatty liver of pregnancy, ulcerative colitis.

B Sonographic features

The liver is enlarged with a generally echogenic appearance. Vascular structures including portal vein walls are less well defined and less prominent than normal and there is usually increased attenuation of the ultrasound beam reducing beam penetration. Changes are inconstant and non-specific.

2.2 CAUSES OF DIFFUSELY INCREASED LIVER ECHOGENICITY

('Bright liver')
Normal variant
Fatty infiltration
Cirrhosis
Diffuse infiltration e.g. glycogen storage
    disease, Gaucher's disease
Miliary granulomata e.g. TB
Extensive malignant infiltration
Infectious mononucleosis
Portal tract fibrosis
Acute alcoholic hepatitis
Severe viral or other hepatitis
Chronic cardiac failure and venous congestion
Hyperalimantation
Malnutrition
Brucellosis
Wilson's disease
Fructose intolerance
Reye's syndrome
Tyrosinaemia
Steroid therapy particularly in conjunction
    with cytotoxic agents
Radiotherapy (majority of cases show no
    detectable change)

2.3 CAUSES OF FOCAL INCREASE IN HEPATIC ECHOGENICITY

Regenerating nodules
Metastases, e.g. bowel or ovary
Primary tumours e.g. haemangioma
Adenoma, focal nodular hyperplasia
Focal fatty infiltration, particularly in alcoholics
  who have recently changed their pattern of
  drinking. Also diabetics. Sonographic
  features may change over a relatively short
  period
Abscess
Infarct
Haematoma/laceration
Hepatitis, particularly CMV and alpha 1
  antitrypsin deficiency
Lipoma/angiomyolipoma

2.3.1 Cirrhosis

Cirrhosis is a pathological condition due to severe liver damage in which the liver shows evidence of both damage and repair. Histologically this is seen as a combination of hepatocyte necrosis and fibrotic scarring with nodules of regenerating liver tissue. These changes distort hepatic architecture further reducing the efficiency of surviving liver tissue. Pathologically cirrhosis may be divided into micro- and macronodular forms depending upon the size of regenerating nodules though in the late stages of cirrhosis the two forms merge as microscopic nodules enlarge. The two commonest causes of cirrhosis are alcoholic liver damage and viral hepatitis.

A Sonographic features

In the early stages of liver damage the liver may be enlarged but it then returns to normal size or shrinks. The caudate lobe is often relatively spared and may appear enlarged. (Caudate lobe is usually half the width of the right lobe measuring from the lateral edge of the caudate lobe to the free edge of each lobe.) In mild cases the liver may appear normal but most advanced cases will show sonographic changes particularly of increased hepatic echogenicity. The hepatic parenchyma appears 'bright' or abnormally echogenic with a fine echotexture. The degree of sonographic abnormality correlates poorly with the degree of liver dysfunction as the latter depends not only upon liver cell necrosis but also upon disordered hepatic architecture and the efficiency of regenerating nodules. Regenerating nodules may give the liver surface an uneven appearance. This may also be seen in cystic fibrosis and malignancy.

Increased hepatic echogenicity reduces the apparent echogenicity of the portal vein walls and may make adjacent renal parenchyma appear relatively hypoechoic. In all cases of suspected hepatic abnormality the portal vein (normal diameter less than 1.5 cm) and splenic vein (normal diameter less than 1 cm/should show alteration in calibre with respiration) should be examined for signs of portal hypertension and the splenic size should be noted. Increased hepatic echogenicity is seen more frequently in micronodular than macronodular cirrhosis though the latter is associated with a greater incidence of hepatoma which may complicate 5 % of cases. Regenerating nodules are rarely seen sonographically and when identified may be indistinguishable from hepatoma.

Ultrasonography is over 80 % accurate at showing

parenchymal abnormality in biopsy proven cases of cirrhosis. However cirrhosis and fatty liver cannot be reliably differentiated sonographically.

2.4 PROMINENT PERIPORTAL ECHOES

Acute cholecystitis
Chronic cholecystitis
Cholangitis
Recurrent pyogenic cholangitis (Oriental
  cholangiohepatitis)
Infectious mononucleosus
Lymphoma
Hepatocellular carcinoma
Periportal fibrosis
Cholangiocarcinoma, particularly Klatskin
  tumours
Cystic fibrosis
Schistosomiasis
Air in the biliary tree (entero-biliary fistula)
  (sphincterotomy)

N.B. Similar appearances may occur with generalized decrease in hepatic echogenicity which make periportal echoes appear relatively more prominent. Reduced renal parenchymal echogenicity may also make assessment of hepatic echotexture difficult.

2.5   INCREASED PERIPORTAL ECHOES IN NEONATES

Acute hepatitis
Cytomegalovirus infection
Biliary atresia
Idiopathic neonatal jaundice
Alpha 1 antitrypsin deficiency
Nesideroblastosis

2.6   CAUSES OF HEPATOMEGALY IN THE NEONATE

Heart failure
Infection
Metastasis
Primary neoplasia
Metabolic defects
Nutritional disorders
Hepatotoxins
Biliary atresia

2.7 NEONATAL LIVER CALCIFICATIONS

Transplacental infection
    Cytomegalovirus
    Herpes
    Toxoplasmosis
Primary and metastatic tumours
    Haemangiomas
    Hamartomas
    Hepatocellular carcinoma
    Hepatoblastoma
Vascular anomalies
    Calcified venous thrombi (particularly post
    umbilical vessel catheterization)
    Haematoma
Abscess
Biliary calcifications

2.8 HEPATIC TUMOURS

Benign hepatic tumours are more common than malignant tumours in neonates and infants, however in adults and older children malignant tumours and metastases are more common. In young children haemangioendothelioma and mesenchymal hamartoma are the two commonest benign tumours.

2.8.1 Haemangioendothelioma

Haemangioendothelioma is the commonest hepatic neoplasm in the neonate. The majority of these tumours present as liver masses in children less than six months old. They are vascular tumours which may be associated with skin haemangiomas in up to 24 % of cases. High blood flow though the tumour may lead to cardiac failure and haemolysis may also occur. They are seen as homogenous masses which are usually echogenic though if the vascular spaces within the tumour are particularly large they may appear hypoechoic. High tumour blood flow may cause dilatation of the aorta and hepatic veins.

2.8.2 Mesenchymal hamartoma

This is the second commonest benign liver tumour in young children. It is seen as a well defined liver mass with some echogenic foci but cystic spaces with septations are more prominent. Malignant mesenchymomas occur but tend to affect older children more than the benign form.

2.8.3 Liver haemangiomas

Liver haemangiomas are the most frequently encountered benign liver tumours, they are usually incidental findings in adults and do not usually cause symptoms or biochemical abnormalities. They can enlarge in pregnancy and uncommonly cause failure to thrive or cardiac failure in children. Sonographically they have a wide range of appearances due to the variation in size of the vascular channels but the most frequent appearance is that of a well defined highly echogenic nodule.

A Capillary haemangiomata

These contain numerous small vessels and are seen as echogenic foci with ill-defined or well-defined margins. They are of variable size but tend to be small and situated superficially within the liver.

B   *Cavernous haemangiomata*

Large sinusoidal vessels give a lobulated hypo- or anechoic appearance though internal echoes may occur and there is usually no distal acoustic enhancement. Hemorrhage into these lesions may occur making appearances complex. Fluid-fluid levels have been recorded and echogenic and complex lesions cannot be reliably differentiated from metastases. Doppler studies may confirm the vascular nature of these lesions and diagnosis may be confirmed at angiography. Biopsy should be avoided as it may cause catastrophic haemorrhage.

Haemangiomas usually show little change in appearance over prolonged periods. Spontaneous regression has been recorded.

2.8.4   Liver adenomas

These uncommon tumours usually occur in adults but may affect children particularly in association with other abnormalities such as glycogen storage disease or Fanconi anaemia. True hepatic adenomas consist of sheets of hepatocytes, other liver cells being absent. They are usually large at the time of diagnosis (5 cm or more) and may cause abdominal pain or haemorrhage. They occur most frequently in women of reproductive age and show a strong link with oestrogens and the contraceptive pill. Sonographic features are variable particularly if the adenoma has been complicated by haemorrhage. The most frequent appearance is of an echogenic mass which is well defined and of relatively uniform appearance though hypoechoic and anechoic areas may be seen. A hypoechoic rim may also be seen. Appearances may be particularly unusual in adenomas associated with an underlying liver abnormality such as glycogen storage disease. In these cases the adenoma may appear poorly defined, hypoechoic and inhomogenous. If the echopattern is similar to that of adjacent liver tissue the adenoma may be difficult to identify.

2.8.5 Biliary cystic adenoma

This rare benign biliary tumour has a complex multicystic mass appearance.

2.8.6 Focal nodular hyperplasia

Hyperplastic nodules of liver parenchyma occurring in focal nodular hyperplasia contain all the normal cellular elements of liver tissue but lack normal hepatic architecture and are thus poorly functioning. This benign condition may occur at any age but is rare in children and is said to occur most frequently in young women. There is no risk of malignant change, though without treatment the lesions may become large. Sonographically, approximately half these lesions appear hypoechoic, nearly half appear echogenic and the remainder have a mixed heterogenous appearance. They are usually well defined lesions and are multiple in 13 % of cases. The majority are vascular on angiography though a small number appear hypovascular. As with liver haemangiomas biopsy should be avoided if possible as there is a risk of haemorrhage.

2.8.7 Hepatic cysts

Though simple liver cysts are seen less frequently than renal cysts they are not uncommon. When multiple they are often associated with cystic disease in other organs. The converse is not true as only 10 % of cases of renal polycystic disease are associated with hepatic cysts. Infantile renal polycystic disease is associated with hepatic fibrosis and not macroscopic cystic disease. Solitary simple hepatic cysts occur in 1 % of the population, their incidence rises with age. When large they may compress bile ducts and liver parenchyma but they are usually asymptomatic. They are seen as spherical or oval anechoic masses. They have a sharp well defined border and give rise to distal acoustic enhancement which may make the posterior border appear prominent. Small cysts may not be detectable as reverberation echoes may make them appear solid. If the cyst wall is prominent or irregular an alternative diagnosis such as abscess, tumour necrosis, hydatid or lymphoma deposit should be considered. Rarely simple cysts may show septae which are usually secondary to trauma and internal haemorrhage.

2.8.8 Malignant hepatic tumours

Hepatoblastoma (51 %) and hepatocellular carcinoma (43 %) are the commonest primary malignant liver tumours in children. Others include rhabdomyosarcoma, teratocarcinoma, angiosarcoma and mesenchymal sarcoma arising from bile ducts and supportive elements within the liver.

2.8.9 Hepatoblastoma

Hepatoblastoma is the commonest primary hepatic malignancy in childhood. The majority of cases present under three years of age usually as an enlarging abdominal mass. Liver function tests are usually normal though the alpha foetoprotein level is elevated in up to 90 % of cases. There is an association with other conditions such as hemi-hypertrophy, macroglossia and sexual precocity. The right lobe of liver is the commonest site for these tumours which are seen as homogenous or heterogenous echogenic masses. Sonolucent foci and isoechoic tumours have been described. Appearances are often non-specific but invasion of vessels may give an indication of the masses malignant nature.

2.8.10   Hepatoma

Hepatoma (hepatocellular carcinoma) is an uncommon tumour in the United Kingdom though there is a remarkable geographic variation in incidence. It is common in the Far East and in black South Africans though it is less common in the rest of Africa and Asia and is uncommon in Americans and Europeans. In adult cases in the United Kingdom 90 % of patients give a history of underlying cirrhosis or other liver disorder. Patients present with right upper quadrant pain or sudden deterioration in hepatic function in an already compromised liver. Rapid local and distant tumour spread results in a poor prognosis with a mean survival of six months from diagnosis. Pathologically a hepatoma may appear nodular, massive or diffuse (infiltrating). Sonographic appearances are similarly variable ranging from cystic to densely echogenic solid masses. The incidence of each appearance varies in each series and there are no pathognmonic appearances. Sonographically a hepatoma may appear identical to extensive metastatic disease and ultrasound guided biopsy may be the most helpful means of confirming the diagnosis. Regenerating nodules may also mimic hepatoma but are generally not as echogenic or heterogenous. Ultrasonography is 95 % accurate at showing a liver abnormality in cases of hepatoma but isoechoic tumours may occur and thus a normal ultrasound scan cannot entirely exclude hepatoma. Early abscess formation may give the liver parenchyma a heterogenous appearance. If liver involvement by infection is extensive infection can mimic massive tumour infiltration. Follow up examination or biopsy may allow diagnosis of these cases.

2.8.11 Rhabdomyosarcoma

This gives rise to a solitary, relatively well defined heterogenous mass of reduced echogenicity. In certain cases cystic spaces with septations may be apparent.

2.8.12 Hepatic metastases

The liver is a very common site for metastases which may be secondary to almost any primary tumour in the body. They are usually multiple but may appear single, particularly if detected early. Multiple metastases give rise to multiple masses within the liver. These often show a range of sizes suggesting that tumour seeding has occurred in episodes. Growing metastases compress adjacent liver parenchyma causing atrophy and forming a connective tissue rim. Large metastases often outgrow their blood supply causing hypoxia and necrosis at the centre of the lesion. The sonographic appearances of metastases are quite variable reflecting the wide spectrum of tumour types. Generally metastases cause hepatomegaly, though this may not be evident until the disease is advanced. Intrahepatic masses may alter hepatic shape and the liver surface may appear nodular. This latter sign is non-specific and also occurs in cystic fibrosis and liver infiltrations.

A Echopatterns

Metastases may be
   Echogenic
   Echopoor
   Iso-echoic
   Mixed (echogenic and echopoor areas)
   Bullseye/target lesion (the centre of the target lesion
      may be hyper- or hypo-echoic)
   Complex (cystic/solid)

These changes may be focal or diffuse. There is relatively poor correlation between the sonographic appearance and tumour histology. Iso-echoic and infiltrating metastases may be particularly difficult to identify.

B Metastases: echopatterns

ECHOGENIC METASTASES – Carcinoma, particularly from gut, pancreas, ovary or hepatoma.

ECHOPOOR METASTASES – Any tumour but particularly homogenous tissue e.g. lymphoma.

CYSTIC METASTASES – Particularly mucin-secreting tumours of ovary, colon, pancreas and stomach. Apparent cystic change may also occur in any metastasis undergoing central necrosis.

CALCIFIED METASTASES – These metastases appear densely echogenic and if calcification is sufficient will give rise to distal acoustic shadowing.

   Aetiology: Carcinoma of colon particularly mucin-secreting type, pseudomucinous cystadenocarcinoma of ovary, adenocarcinoma of stomach and rarely adenocarcinoma of breast or melanoma. In children neuroblastoma is the commonest metastasis, it is usually hypoechoic but may show calcification and can be echogenic.

Tumours responding to therapy may show increased echogenicity but more often show decreased size with central necrosis.

C 'Bulls eye' appearance in hepatic mass lesions in children

Tumours e.g. hepatocellular carcinoma
metastasis from bowel tumour
liver adenoma in glycogen storage disease
abscesses including fungal abscess

D Diffuse malignancy

Diffuse hepatic malignancy is seen less frequently than focal disease. Diffuse disease may be due to confluence of areas of focal disease, infiltrating tumours or miliary metastatic deposits. The liver may appear 'moth eaten' with a patchy echopattern which may be of increased or decreased echogenicity, or, uncommonly, the infiltrates are isoechoic.

Lymphoma and leukaemia are particularly prone to diffuse disease which usually appears hypoechoic though these changes do not always reflect the presence of metastases as reactive lymphocytic infiltration secondary to disease elsewhere may give rise to the same appearance. When the liver is extensively replaced by metastases jaundice may occur due to inadequate liver function. Alternatively Hodgkins disease may cause intrahepatic biliary obstruction at the canalicular level whilst lymphadenopathy may compress the extrahepatic biliary system. Even in the absence of jaundice liver function tests usually show some abnormality in the presence of metastatic disease.

2.8.13   Hepatic trauma

Injury of the abdominal viscera may be due to blunt abdominal trauma or penetrating wounds. The solid organs and retroperitoneal segments of bowel are more prone to injury than bowel suspended on a mesentery as the latter is more mobile. Liver injury occurs more easily in children than in adults as the ribs are more flexible allowing a force to be transmitted to the liver. Also the liver is not fully developed, having a weaker connective tissue framework than in adults. Trauma may cause acute or delayed haemorrhage with parenchymal laceration. An expanding haematoma may lead to delayed liver rupture and resolving haematomas may give rise to hepatic cysts. In addition laceration of the biliary system may lead to the formation of biliary fistulas or bile collections.

During active haemorrhage, blood is anechoic though there is less distal acoustic enhancement behind a newly formed haematoma than posterior to a bile collection. As the blood clots the haematoma changes, becoming echogenic with a heterogenous pattern. Later the clot breaks down and liquefies forming anechoic areas giving a complex cystic appearance. Fluid/debris and fluid/fluid levels have been reported within resolving haematomas. Chronic persistence of a fluid collection after trauma suggests other complications such as cyst or biloma formation.

2.8.14   Hepatic infection

Focal infection of the liver parenchyma is an uncommon but potentially fatal condition and thus a high index of suspicion is required if it is to be diagnosed sufficiently early to allow successful treatment. Hepatic infection occurs more frequently in adults than children and may complicate any infective process. The majority of infections are pyogenic and reach the liver either via the hepatic artery during septicaemia, via the portal vein from abdominal infection or via the biliary tree in ascending cholangitis.

2.8.15 Pyogenic liver abscess

Pyogenic liver abscesses are uncommon in children. The majority of these cases occur in the under five age group and may occur secondary to umbilical vein catheterization, appendicitis, surgery, renal infection or immune deficiency such as chronic granulomatous disease of childhood. In older children the infection is often with staphylococci whilst in adults 50 % of infections are anaerobic reflecting the frequency of spread of infection from bowel. Sonographic appearances are very variable reflecting not only the nature and extent of infection but also the stage of abscess formation. Initially as the infection involves the liver appearances are normal then subtle parenchymal changes occur, usually a reduction in echogenicity. As tissue inflammation progresses an area of increased or decreased echogenicity forms which may be quite heterogenous. Necrosis and pus formation at the centre of the abscess gives rise to an anechoic or hypoechoic area with few internal echoes, an irregular wall and variable distal acoustic enhancement. Established abscesses may contain debris or uncommonly appear septate. A hypoechoic rim may surround the outer margin of the abscess. As a fibrous reaction occurs around the abscess an increasingly echogenic wall forms which may calcify in longstanding cases giving very high level echoes with or without distal acoustic shadowing.

Gas-forming organisms may give rise to intense echoes arising in the centre of the abscess rather than in the wall. If the abscess is successfully treated with antibiotics but without surgical or radiological drainage then follow up will show slow reduction in the size of the anechoic collection with increasing organization of the echogenic wall which may leave a permanent scar.

2.8.16 Fungal liver abscess

Focal fungal liver abscess is quite uncommon and usually occurs in immune-suppressed patients particularly during chemotherapy for cancer such as leukaemia. Fungal abscesses are usually multiple being seen as multiple hypoechoic areas or less often as multiple target lesions which may be indistinguishable from multiple metastases.

2.8.17 Hydatid liver disease

Infection with the cystic stage of the tapeworm *Echinococcus granulosus* results in hydatid disease. This affects the liver in two-thirds of cases. In endemic areas over 95 % of the population show positive serological evidence of infection. In the United Kingdom infection is usually found in patients who have lived abroad or in sheep-rearing areas as sheep, like man, is an intermediate host for the tapeworm.

A Sonographic features of liver hydatids
  Simple fluid filled cyst. This is the earliest appearance and is usually indistinguishable from a simple cyst
  Cyst with undulating membranes. Undulating membranes occur within the cyst due to endocyst rupture

Cysts within a cyst. Due to the presence of daughter
  cysts within a larger cyst

Multilocular cyst with echogenic matrix material.
  If the echogenic matrix predominates then the
  hydatid may appear solid

Complex mass with cystic and solid areas

Densely calcified mass with distal shadowing

Heterogenous mass with areas of increased and
  decreased echogenicity. This is usually due to
  secondary infection. If air is present the lesion
  may be very echogenic

Hydatid cysts are usually round or oval, well defined
and usually have a demonstrable wall. Though diagnosis
is straightforward in typical cases many hydatids have
non-specific appearances and serological tests for hydatid infection should be performed prior to biopsy of a
possible lesion. (Biopsy is to be avoided in hydatids
owing to the risk of spreading infection.)

2.8.18 Echinococcus multilocularis

Infection with the tapeworm *Echinococcus multilocularis* results in a solid heterogenous appearance far
more commonly than granulosus infection. Fine echogenic areas may give the resulting mass a 'hail storm'
appearance. The resulting mass may have a nodular
appearance with cystic and necrotic areas. Calcification
may also occur. Infection may be associated with portal
hypertension, portal vein thrombosis, IVC thrombosis,
splenic or retroperitoneal disease.

2.8.19 Schistosomiasis

The freshwater snail acts as intermediate host in
infection. Cercaria penetrate the skin and reach the

liver, gut and bladder via the blood stream. Here they promote a granulomatous reaction causing hepatic fibrosis and cirrhosis. Portal veins show thickening of their walls which are more echogenic than normal. Portal vein deformity results in portal hypertension with splenomegaly and varices.

2.8.20 Hepatic amoebiasis

The protozoan parasite *Entamoeba histolytica* enters the body by ingestion of its cystic form. This may pass through the stomach as the cysts are resistant to acid. The amoebae then colonize the bowel, particularly the caecum and secrete proteolytic enzymes which cause mucosal ulceration. Some amoebae penetrate the bowel wall and reach the liver via the portal venous system. Amoebae may lie dormant in the liver for many years and there is usually a long delay between the initial bowel infection and the clinical presentation of an amoebic liver abscess.

Amoebic abscesses occur most frequently in the right lobe of liver, usually in the superior aspect close to the diaphragm. They are usually single with a thick irregular wall and contain necrotic liver tissue. They may rupture into the subphrenic or subhepatic spaces and may even penetrate the diaphragm to reach the pleural cavity. With successful treatment abscesses resolve leaving an area of focal scarring though old amoebic abscesses may rarely calcify.

Ultrasonography cannot accurately differentiate amoebic and other liver abscesses. The abscess is seen as an anechoic or hypoechoic collection with a thick irregular wall. Occasionally a fluid/debris level may be present.

2.9 CAUSES OF APPARENT HEPATOMEGALY ON CLINICAL EXAMINATION

True hepatomegaly

Riedel's lobe

Downward displacement e.g. pulmonary over-inflation, pleural effusion, subphrenic collection

Masses confused with liver e.g. renal mass, adrenal mass, para-aortic mass/lymph nodes, pancreatic mass/pseudocyst, ascites.

A Hepatic size

Measured at the midpoint between the centre of the spine and the extreme right margin of the right lobe of liver the normal longitudinal measurement is usually less than or equal to 13 cm.

2.10 HEPATIC PSEUDO-LESIONS/PSEUDO-MASS LESIONS

Focal fatty infiltration. Seen as a focal area of increased echogenicity with angulated margins and interdigitation with normal liver tissue

Focal areas of reduced echogenicity at the porta hepatis. Irregular ovoid or spherical areas of reduced echogenicity may be due to focal sparing in fatty infiltration

Hypoechoic caudate lobe. This is a normal variant due to acoustic shadowing by fibrous tissue in the ligamentum venosum

Hypoechoic quadrate lobe. A sign of generalized fatty infiltration

Falciform ligament. This is the commonest echogenic pseudolesion in the liver

Perihepatic fat. Normal variation in the amount of intra-abdominal fat and its distribution in relation to the liver borders may cause indentation of the hepatic margin simulating disease. This is seen most frequently between the liver and right kidney and between the left lobe and chest wall

Air in the biliary tree, e.g. post sphincterotomy usually has a linear echogenic branching pattern which may be mistaken for calcification or even metastases

Diaphragm leaflets. May appear to interdigitate with the liver particularly with a broad ultrasound beam

The lateral aspect of the left lobe of liver may lie adjacent to or just above the medial aspect of the spleen and may be mistaken for a hypoechoic mass such as an abscess or haematoma

2.11 MULTISEPTATE CYSTIC HEPATIC MASS LESIONS

Metastases e.g. pancreas, ovary, stomach, colon, bronchus. May be from a primarily cystic tumour or necrosis within a large metastasis. This is the commonest cause in our clinical practice

Infective cysts e.g. hydatid cysts, pyogenic abscess; amoebic abscesses

Benign cysts, particularly after internal haemorrhage or infection, hepatic polycystic disease

Traumatic or haemorrhagic cyst

Biliary cyst (also post trauma)

Biliary cystadenoma

Hepatic hamartoma

Mesenchymoma

Teratoma

Cavernous haemangioma

Cystic hepatoblastoma

Infantile peliosis hepatis

2.12 ANECHOIC/HYPOECHOIC INTRAHEPATIC MASSES

Congenital cyst

Post traumatic cyst. May contain internal echoes

Hydatid cyst

Metastasis. Parenchyma around the anechoic area may be abnormal

Primary hepatic tumour

Focal hepatitis

Focal hepatic necrosis. Margins irregular, may have internal echoes and abnormal adjacent parenchyma

Abscess

Haematoma. Anechoic during acute haemorrhage and during clot liquefaction

Biloma. May be post-traumatic

Caroli's disease. Multiple small dilated bile ducts

Extra medullary haematopoiesis

Focal sparing in fatty infiltration

2.12.1 The hepatic artery

The hepatic artery is a branch of the coeliac axis which is a short arterial trunk arising from the anterior surface of the aorta. Less frequently it may arise from the superior mesenteric artery or directly from the aorta. In transverse section the coeliac axis is seen to have a 'seagull' or 'T' configuration. The hepatic artery is very variable in its extrahepatic course. The right branch of the hepatic artery crosses anterior to the portal vein and as it does so it lies between the portal vein and

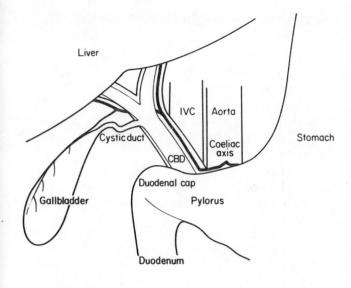

━━Hepatic artery

Fig. 10. Relations of the hepatic artery and biliary system.

common hepatic duct in 80 % of people (Fig. 10). In 15 % it crosses anterior to both common hepatic duct and portal vein.

A Hepatic artery aneurysm/pseudoaneurysm

The hepatic artery is the fourth most frequent site of intra-abdominal arterial aneurysm. Eighty per cent rupture with severe haemorrhage. Pseudo-aneurysms occur when the artery is involved by a local inflammatory process such as pancreatitis.

Sonography shows a non-pulsatile anechoic mass with irregular echogenic walls. Doppler studies show turbulent arterial flow.

2.12.2 Hepatic veins

Superior veins (right, middle and left) drain most of the liver, they are normally up to 1 cm in diameter and pass obliquely backwards to the IVC. Inferior veins drain the caudate lobe and part of the right lobe. Separate caudate lobe venous drainage may allow preservation of caudate lobe function in hepatic vein obstruction (Budd–Chiari syndrome).

2.13 HEPATIC VEIN DISTENSION

Congestive cardiac failure. The IVC is also distended and shows loss of its normal variation in calibre with respiration. The liver may be enlarged

Tricuspid atresia/stenosis

Tumour within right atrium, IVC or invading hepatic veins

Clot within the hepatic venous system

Constrictive pericarditis

A Sonographic features of the Budd–Chiari syndrome

In normal patients at least one of the three main hepatic veins is usually visible. In the Budd–Chiari syndrome (hepatic vein occlusion) the hepatic veins may not be visible or may appear thick-walled, irregular, with areas of stenoses, proximal dilatation, intraluminal thrombus and intrahepatic collaterals. In long-standing cases there is atrophy of the right lobe of liver with hypertrophy of the caudate and lateral segments of the left lobe. The IVC may be compressed by the swollen liver or may be obstructed by clot or tumour. The IVC may show an 'hour glass' configuration in cases associated with coarctation of the IVC. Doppler studies show reduced flow with loss of the normal flow changes with the cardiac cycle.

2.14 THE PORTAL VENOUS SYSTEM

The portal vein is formed behind the neck of pancreas by the fusion of the splenic and superior mesenteric veins. It passes behind the first part of the duodenum to enter the free edge of the lesser omentum with the CBD and hepatic artery. At the porta hepatis it divides into right and left branches which supply the right and left lobes of liver. The portal vein receives the left gastric and superior pancreaticoduodenal veins near the pancreatic head. The cystic vein draining the gallbladder enters the right branch of the portal vein at the porta hepatis. Variations in portal venous anatomy are rare and are usually associated with major anomalies such as malrotation and situs inversus.

2.14.1 Sonographic features of portal hypertension

The majority of cases of portal hypertension are secondary to liver disease which may show sonographic changes. There is dilatation of the portal vein, superior mesenteric vein and splenic vein. The maximum normal portal vein diameter is approximately 1.3 cm. More significantly, the splenic and superior mesenteric veins usually show variation in calibre with respiration. This calibre variation is lost in over 90 % of cases when these veins become distended. (Normally SMV and splenic vein diameter may increase 50–100 % during inspiration.) Splenic and superior mesenteric veins should measure less than 1 cm in diameter.

A Demonstration of portosystemic anastomoses

Oesophageal varices. Seen as anechoic tubes around the oesophagus behind the left lobe of liver

Dilated veins along the course of the umbilical vein and around the umbilicus. The umbilical vein remnant forms part of the ligamentum teres. The umbilical vein is seldom patent except in cases of portal hypertension when it may give rise to a bulls-eye appearance, the anechoic vein being highlighted by the echogenic ligament

Dilated veins in the retroperitoneum

Anastomoses also occur around the rectum but these are usually not visible sonographically

Lieno-renal anastomoses

2.14.2 Splenomegaly

A Ascites

Uncomplicated portal hypertension does not usually cause ascites. Ascites usually occurs secondary to underlying liver disease with liver cell failure.

B Demonstrable portal vein occlusion

The majority of cases of portal hypertension are due to liver disease but a small number of cases are secondary to portal vein occlusion. This is usually due to tumour or thrombus. Non-visualization of the portal vein is strongly suspicious of occlusion. The portal vein may then be seen as a band of high-level echoes at the porta hepatis. Numerous small vessels giving the appearance of multiple fine threads at the porta hepatis indicate cavernous transformation of the portal vein or the formation of collateral vascular channels. Cavernous transformation of the portal vein has been recorded as giving the appearance of a sub-hepatic 'sponge-like' mass. This appearance has also been reported in cases of pancreatic haemangiosarcoma.

2.14.3 Portal vein thrombosis

Failure to visualize the portal vein lumen. (Not due to overlying bowel gas or technical factors.) Failure to demonstrate normal portal vein divisions

Empty porta hepatis – appears as a diamond shaped area of high level echoes

Echogenic thrombus demonstrated within the portal vein lumen

Combination of abdominal mass with intraluminal portal vein clot is strongly suggestive of abdominal malignancy

Enlargement of thrombosed segment of portal vein

Multiple worm-like vascular channels in the porta hepatis due to cavernous transformation of the portal vein. This occurs in longstanding cases and is usually associated with benign disease

Longstanding cases may show evidence of portal hypertension

The hepatic artery may be hypertrophied

Thrombosis is usually secondary to liver disease and portal hypertension but may also occur with hepatic malignancy such as hepatoma or rarely primary leiomyosarcoma may arise in the portal vein.

2.14.4 Portal venous gas

Gas within the portal venous system may occur secondary to bowel ischaemia, infarction, necrotizing enterocolitis and other inflammatory conditions which reduce mucosal integrity or increase intraluminal pressure. Microbubbles are seen as tiny echogenic particles within the portal blood which move with the flow. The gas is rapidly carried peripherally within the intrahepatic portal vein branches and tends to collect in the uppermost branches (left lobe and anterior segment of the right lobe). Collections of gas are then seen as highly echogenic lines which may shadow.

2.15 LIVER ATROPHY WITH COMPENSATORY HYPERTROPHY

Surgical resection
Cirrhosis
Hepatic vein obstruction
Intra-hepatic biliary obstruction e.g.
    intrahepatic cholelithiasis
Cholangiocarcinoma
Radiation therapy
Liver metastases e.g. breast, colon, bile duct,
    squamous cell, tonsillar ca., renal
    transitional cell
Post chemotherapy for hepatic tumour
Budd–Chiari syndrome
Lobar agenesis

2.15.1 The biliary system

The right and left hepatic ducts unite at the porta hepatis to form the common hepatic duct which enters the free edge of the lesser omentum. It is joined by the cystic duct forming the common bile duct (CBD). The CBD is approximately 8 cm long. It lies in the free edge of the lesser omentum, usually situated anterolateral to the portal vein. It then passes behind the superior part of the second part of duodenum and head of pancreas to end at the duodenal papilla. Behind the duodenum the CBD lies anterior to the portal vein with the gastroduodenal artery on its left side. Behind the head of pancreas the CBD lies on the IVC, at this point it receives the common pancreatic duct and turns to the right to enter the duodenum.

2.15.2 Signs of intra-hepatic biliary dilatation

Only the major intra-hepatic biliary radicles are normally visible. These are seen adjacent to the portal vein branches close to the porta hepatis. Visualization of smaller bile ducts within the liver is always abnormal.

A *Signs of biliary dilatation*

Parallel channel sign. In longitudinal section, two anechoic tubes are seen side by side. The tube with the echogenic walls is a portal vein branch, the dilated bile duct does not have visible walls

Double-barrel shotgun sign. In transverse section the dilated bile duct and adjacent portal vein branch are seen as two adjacent anechoic circles

Too many tubes. The sonographer gets the impression that there are too many tubular structures in the liver. These tubes have a stellate configuration radiating from the porta

Dilated ducts are often beaded and tortuous

Dilated bile ducts cause less sound attenuation than adjacent blood filled veins. Focal areas of acoustic enhancement may thus be seen behind dilated bile ducts. This may make assessment of liver parenchyma difficult

2.15.3 CBD dimensions

The upper limit of normal for the CBD diameter is usually taken as 0.6 cm but the normal CBD is frequently much smaller than this.

Common hepatic duct. Average diameter at the porta hepatis. 0.25 cm ± 0.11 cm

Common bile duct. Average diameter 0.28 cm ± 0.12 cm

In 95 % of patients the normal CBD is equal to or less than 0.4 cm.

Post cholecystectomy CHD and CBD dimensions are generally slightly greater than prior to surgery – CHD mean diameter 0.52 cm ± 0.23 cm at the porta and CBD 0.62 cm ± 0.25 cm. Patients with gallstones also tend to have larger extra-hepatic bile ducts though this does not always mean that there are gallstones within the bile ducts at the time of examination. Average duct diameter at the widest point of the CBD in patients with gallstones is 0.48 cm ± 0.22 cm.

2.15.4 Biliary obstruction

The upper limit of normal for the serum bilirubin level is around 17 μM l^{-1} but patients with elevated serum bilirubin do not become visibly jaundiced until the serum bilirubin level exceeds 30 μM l^{-1}. Increased serum bilirubin may occur secondary to increased red cell breakdown, hepatocellular dysfunction or obstruction to biliary drainage. These groups are not clearly defined as any longstanding biliary obstruction may cause hepatocellular damage which may cause persistent jaundice even after biliary obstruction has been relieved.

Dilatation of the biliary tree usually precedes biochemical evidence of biliary obstruction and jaundice. The degree of biliary dilatation depends upon the degree of obstruction, the speed of onset and the duration. In sudden, complete obstruction dilatation may take a week to occur but generally in patients with established jaundice lack of biliary dilatation excludes the diagnosis of major bile duct obstruction. It should be remembered that lymphadenopathy at the porta hepatis may cause biliary obstruction without visible dilatation of the extra-hepatic ducts and a biochemical picture of obstructive jaundice may occur due to intra-hepatic obstruction at a canalicular level.

Biliary manometry performed at percutaneous transhepatic cholangiography shows an almost linear relationship between bile duct diameter and biliary pressure. The normal intraduct pressure is between 5 and 18 cm of water. This close relation between bile duct size and pressure makes ultrasonography a reliable means for the detection of extrahepatic biliary obstruction but sonography is less reliable at determining the level and cause of obstruction. When doubt exists about the state of the biliary system a repeat examination after a short delay may be invaluable.

2.15.5 Patterns of biliary dilatation

A Dilatation of peripheral radicles

The major intra-hepatic bile ducts may be visible near the porta hepatis but the remaining intra-hepatic ducts are not normally seen. When intra-hepatic bile ducts are dilated they become visible and are seen as serpiginous tubes which lie directly adjacent to the portal vein branches. Bile causes less attenuation of the ultrasound beam than blood in the adjacent veins and soft tissues thus distal acoustic enhancement may be evident. Dilated ducts seen in transverse section have a 'double-barrel' appearance due to the adjacent portal venous radicle.

B   Dilatation of the common hepatic duct

The point of union of the cystic duct and common hepatic duct cannot be exactly defined on ultrasonography and thus the point of transition from common hepatic duct to common bile duct cannot be accurately demarcated. The common hepatic duct is seen antero-lateral to the portal vein in the porta hepatis. The right branch of the hepatic artery is frequently seen passing between these two structures. The upper limit of normal for CHD diameter is 4 mm. CHD dilatation is not always associated with intrahepatic bile duct dilatation particularly in early cases of biliary obstruction.

C   Common bile duct dilatation

The dilated common bile duct lies antero-lateral to the portal vein. When examining the patient with the right side elevated three adjacent tubular structures may be seen. These are CBD, portal vein and IVC from anterior to posterior. The distal CBD may be obscured by bowel gas as it passes behind the duodenum but an attempt should be made to identify the most distal point of duct dilatation. The normal CBD is up to 6 mm in diameter though post cholecystectomy it may be up to 10 mm.

D　*Gallbladder dilatation*

This is an unreliable sign of biliary obstruction as

> The normal gallbladder can show marked enlargement when a patient is fasting
>
> Some patients with frank obstruction show only slight gallbladder distension
>
> A diseased gallbladder may be incapable of contraction or distension

2.16　BILIARY DILATATION WITHOUT JAUNDICE

> Early obstruction
>
> Post obstruction
>
> Gallstones. Either within the gallbladder or within the CBD but without acute obstruction
>
> Post cholecystectomy
>
> Intraluminal sludge ball e.g. in severe haemolysis
>
> Only part of biliary system obstructed
>
> Worms/parasites
>
> Normal variant. This diagnosis should be made with extreme caution after exclusion of other causes and prolonged follow up
>
> Age. CBD calibre increases with age and upper limit of normal may be 0.75 cm at 75 years

2.17 BILIARY OBSTRUCTION WITHOUT APPARENT DILATATION

Sudden severe biliary obstruction
Biliary fibrosis e.g. post sclerosing cholangitis, this may prevent dilatation of obstructed ducts
Cholangitis
Small calculi
Pancreatitis
Haemobilia
Ducts filled with debris
Cholangiocarcinoma ⎱ Tumour
Metastases ⎰ encasement
Previous surgery in this area (fibrosis)
Technical difficulties giving poor visualization

2.18 BILIARY OBSTRUCTION IN THE NEWBORN

Extra-hepatic biliary atresia
Intra-hepatic biliary atresia with/without lymphoedema
Bile duct hypoplasia
Bile plug syndrome
Choledochal cyst
Cystic fibrosis
Biliary/hepatic neoplasms
Periductal lymphoedema

2.19 COMMON HEPATIC DUCT DILATATION

Upper limit of normal – 4 mm

Post cholecystectomy upper limit of normal – 7 mm

Choledochal cyst/choledochocoele

Calculus

Choledochal diverticulum

Mirizzi syndrome. (CHD obstruction due to a stone impacted in the cystic duct)

Oriental cholangio-hepatitis. (There may be a large amount of sludge in the duct with or without stones)

Primary or secondary cholangitis

Cholangiocarcinoma

Any cause of CBD dilatation e.g. carcinoma of the head of pancreas

Compression by lymph nodes

AIDS

2.20 INTRALUMINAL CBD MASS

Calculus
Sludge/debris
Blood clot
Cholangiocarcinoma
Adenocarcinoma
Food/faeces (entero-biliary fistula)
Worms/parasites e.g. *Ascaris lumbricoides*
Intraductal hepatoma
Pus

2.20.1 Neonatal jaundice

Persistent or increasing jaundice in the late neonatal period is a worrying problem because of the risk of underlying biliary atresia. Early diagnosis and surgical treatment are essential if permanent liver damage is to be reduced to a minimum. The main differential diagnosis in these cases is biliary atresia or neonatal hepatitis. Neonatal hepatitis may occur due to

Idiopathic (majority)
Infection e.g. CMV or other virus
Cholestasis e.g. alpha 1 antitrypsin deficiency
    arteriohepatic dysplasia, Byler's disease

A *Sonographic features of neonatal hepatitis*

The liver and biliary system may appear normal
Bile ducts are of normal calibre though appearances of the gallbladder are variable and it may not be visible
Hepatic echogenicity is often normal at presentation but may be increased in longstanding cases

2.20.2 Biliary atresia

Biliary atresia may take one of several forms:

Diffuse extrahepatic biliary atresia (commonest). Probably due to chronic cholangitis *in utero*

Focal atresia. Probably due to intrauterine vascular insult. This form is more amenable to treatment than the other types

Intra-hepatic duct atresia. May be due to intrauterine infection such as reovirus.

A *Sonographic features*

Initially the liver shows slight enlargement. Hepatic echogenicity may be normal or may be heterogenous and increased. The presence of a visible gallbladder reduces the likelihood of biliary atresia but does not exclude it. Gallbladder contraction after a fatty meal is presumptive evidence of biliary drainage but may not occur in cases of neonatal hepatitis thus absence of gallbladder contraction does not shorten the differential diagnosis.

Biliary atresia is uncommon affecting 1 in 20 000 live births but should always be considered in cases of neonatal jaundice as the complications of delayed diagnosis are severe. Though ultrasonography is valuable in the assessment of the biliary system dilated ducts are not evident in extra-hepatic biliary atresia and a Tc 99m HIDA isotope scan is a valuable means of demonstrating biliary drainage. Severe cases of neonatal hepatitis may also show abnormalities of biliary drainage due to bile stasis and all such cases should have further assessment of the biliary system by laparoscopy or chalangiography. Bile formation occurs from the 12th week of intrauterine life. The

earlier that biliary atresia occurs *in utero* the greater
the liver damage that occurs before birth. Thus, despite
early diagnosis and intervention some cases have irreversible liver damage at presentation.

2.20.3   Choledochal cyst

Choledochal cysts are a form of cystic dilatation of the
biliary system. These cysts may be classified by their
anatomy (Fig. 11). Type:

1) Localized cystic dilatation of the CBD. CHD,
   cystic duct and gallbladder are normal. (Commonest form)
2) Choledochal cyst is a diverticulum arising from
   the CBD
3) Choledochal cyst is an invagination of the CBD
   (choledochocoele) into the duodenum analogous
   to a ureterocoele in the bladder
4) Dilatation of the whole CBD and CHD

Choledochal cysts usually present with an abdominal
mass, pain, fever or jaundice. The latter is only present
in 42 % and only 25 % give a classic history. The
incidence of cysts is greatest in children but they may
occur in adults and may be associated with gallstones,
pancreatitis or even cirrhosis. However, the majority
of cases are thought to be congenital in origin due to
bile reflux. Eight per cent of cases are associated with
Caroli's disease.

A   Sonographic features

The cysts are seen as anechoic fluid filled structures in
the right upper quadrant though their communication
with the biliary tree may not be apparent. Remaining
biliary system may be dilated but despite this choledo-

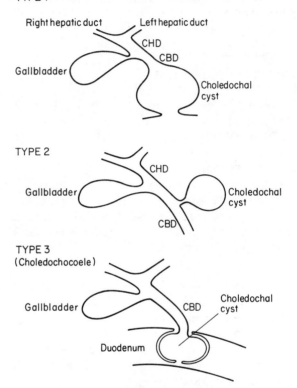

Fig. 11. Choledochal cysts.

chal cysts may be indistinguishable from other upper abdominal cysts. The diagnosis may be confirmed with a HIDA isotope scan which usually (but not always) shows accumulation of tracer within the cyst.

2.21   CHOLEDOCHAL CYST: DIFFERENTIAL DIAGNOSIS

Hepatic cyst
Pancreatic pseudocyst
Enteric duplication cyst
Hepatic artery aneurysm
Spontaneous perforation of the biliary system

A   Sonographic features of Klatskin tumours

Bile duct carcinomas are rare. They are usually associated with gallstones, inflammatory bowel disease or cystic disease of the biliary tree. Ten to twenty-five per cent of bile-duct carcinomas arise at the porta hepatis and are then called Klatskin tumours. Most are adenocarcinomas but squamous carcinomas also occur. They tend to grow slowly.

FEATURES –

Dilatation of intra-hepatic bile ducts without extrahepatic duct dilatation
Lack of communication of left and right major intrahepatic bile ducts
Usually no evidence of ductal calculi but frequently associated with stones within the gallbladder
Normal pancreas
Invasion of adjacent liver
No other known primary tumour
   79 % are echogenic
   19 % are hypoechoic
   2 % have a mixed echopattern

2.21.1   Caroli's disease

This is a rare syndrome in which there is non-obstructive saccular dilatation of the intrahepatic bile ducts. This is associated with an increased incidence of biliary stones, cholangitis and biliary cirrhosis. Some cases are also associated with congential hepatic fibrosis and autosomal recessive renal polycystic disease. Caroli's disease is thought to be a form of congenital biliary ectasia but usually presents in adults. It is more common in females than males. Ultrasonography shows irregular dilatation of intrahepatic bile ducts without obvious extrahepatic cause such as nodes at the porta. Small intra-duct stones and gallstones may also be evident. Portal vein radicles may appear entirely surrounded by dilated bile ducts which may show 'bridge' formation across the lumina.

2.21.2 Worms and parasites

Worms and parasites may enter the biliary and pancreatic ducts from the duodenum. Though worms are seldom seen in the biliary system in the United Kingdom worm infestation is a world wide problem and should be considered in cases of atypical biliary dilatation. *Ascaris lumbricoides* is the worm most frequently seen in the biliary tract. It gives rise to linear intra-duct filling defects which do not shadow unless dead and calcified. In transverse section they have a 'bulls eye' appearance due to their echogenic walls and anechoic centre. Multiple worms have been reported as giving the appearance of overlapping tubes or spaghetti. Adult worms may grow to up to 30 cm in length and 0.5 cm in diameter.

2.21.3 Pneumobilia

Pneumobilia is the presence of air within the biliary tree. This is usually due to air ascending from the duodenum but may rarely be due to cholangitis. Ascending air is seen most frequently after ERCP and sphincterotomy but may also occur after the passage of gallstones or distortion of the lower CBD by local inflammation, tumour or duodenal ulceration. Air within the biliary tree is seen as densely echogenic lines with shadowing along the course of the biliary system. The air is not carried peripherally to the same extent as portal venous gas.

2.21.4 Spontaneous biliary perforation

This is an uncommon condition but is the second commonest surgical cause of jaundice in the newborn. It also occurs in adults when it is usually secondary to inflammation or gallstones.

A Aetiology

Trauma
Biliary obstruction
Biliary stones
Congenital anomaly with reflux of pancreatic fluid
Congenital wall weaknesses
Congenital wall ischaemia

In children the leak is usually at the junction of the CBD and cystic duct. This results in a subacute illness with jaundice, pale stools and abdominal distension. Less often it may present as an acute fulminating hepatitis. On sonography the biliary system may appear normal but there is usually ascites or a local collection. A HIDA scan will confirm the bile leak by showing tracer spreading around the peritoneal cavity. In adults biliary rupture due to gallstones presents as a more acute illness with peritonitis.

2.21.5 The gallbladder

The gallbladder is a pear-shaped sac lying in the gallbladder bed posteromedial to the right lobe of liver. The fundus of the gallbladder is usually close to the anterior abdominal wall in the region of the ninth costal cartilage. At this point it is covered by peritoneum and is adjacent to the hepatic flexure of colon which may obscure it. The body of gallbladder is adjacent to the duodenum which indents it and may mimic gallstones or a gallbladder mass. The mucosa of the gallbladder neck is thrown into folds giving an echogenic appearance which may also mimic gallstones. A small pouch projects from the right side of the gallbladder neck. This is Hartmann's pouch which when visible is frequently associated with pathology particularly dilatation. The gallbladder fundus is often 'folded over' and the gallbladder then assumes a double-barrel appearance.

2.21.6 Gallbladder dimensions

The average gallbladder measures:

Length 7–10 cm (the normal gallbladder is nearly always less than 13 cm long)
Diameter 3 cm (less than 4 cm)

In the fasting patient the normal gallbladder seldom exceeds

4 × 10 cm
Cystic duct length 3–4 cm

Gallbladder size generally increases with age but wall thickness is unaffected by age.

2.21.7 Neonatal gallbladder

Diameter 0.5–1.6 cm mean – 0.9 cm
Average length 2.5 cm
Wall thickness ≤ 1 mm

2.21.8 Adult gallbladder

Wall thickness 0.2 cm or less
Gallbladder volume = (length × width × height)

$$\times \frac{\pi}{6}$$

Simple measurement of gallbladder area in a single plane is usually adequate for the comparison of pre- and post-prandial gallbladder sizes.

Non-visualization of the gallbladder in a truly fasting patient is highly suggestive of gallbladder disease. (At least 88 % have gallbladder pathology with an obliterated lumen.) In some centres oral cholecystography is used as a further imaging modality in these cases. If the ultrasound scan is repeated with further fasting the contracted gallbladder can often be identified.

2.22 GALLBLADDER ANOMALIES

Situs inversus. Gallbladder in the left upper
    quadrant
Gallbladder related to the left side of the liver
    – rare
Heterotaxia. Intermediate situs with the
    gallbladder in the midline. Associated with
    asplenia, polysplenia, pulmonary isomerism
    and congenital heart disease
Unusual gallbladder location e.g. suprahepatic
    in the falciform ligament, intrahepatic or
    retroperitoneal
Free floating pendular gallbladder
Anomalies of shape e.g. phrygian cap –
    gallbladder cap folded back on itself,
    septate gallbladder – this appearance is
    usually due to gallbladder folding
Agenesis. This rare anomaly may be
    associated with biliary atresia, CHD and
    CBD anomalies. Rarely the gallbladder
    opens separately into the duodenum.
Fish hook or hourglass configuration
Gallbladder duplication with two cystic ducts
Heterotopic gastric or pancreatic tissue in the
    gallbladder wall

2.22.1 Gallstones

Gallstones are common, affecting 15 % of the adult
population. They occur more frequently in females
than males. The incidence of gallstones increases with
age though they are not rare in children, particularly
those who have had intravenous feeding. (In these
cases the gallstones may actually resolve.) Chronic

haemolysis such as hereditary spherocytosis and the haemoglobinopathies also predispose to gallstone formation. Up to 27 % of children and 70 % of adults with sickle cell anaemia have gallstones. Ten per cent of gallstones contain sufficient calcium to be visible on plain abdominal radiographs.

A Diagnostic criteria

Mobile echogenic structures with distal acoustic shadowing within the gallbladder lumen on images taken in two planes at right angles – virtually 100 % accurate for gallstones.

Non-visualization of the gallbladder lumen with echogenic structures with distal acoustic shadowing arising in the gallbladder fossa – 96 % accurate for gallstones in a diseased gallbladder.

Gallstones 3 mm or more in diameter usually cause shadowing. The shadowing is 'clean' unlike the shadowing distal to bowel gas which contains reverberation echoes. Reverberation artefact can also occur distal to gallstones but is usually more regular than distal to bowel gas and may give rise to the 'comet tail' appearance which may be related to the calcium content of the stone.

Gallstones usually lie in the most dependent part of the gallbladder but can float in the bile particularly after cholecystographic contrast. It is important that a patient being examined for gallstones is turned from side to side during the examination or small stones which do not cause shadowing may be hidden by the mucosal folds of the spiral valve of Heister.

2.23 CAUSES OF GALLSTONES IN CHILDREN

Haemolysis e.g. hereditary spherocytosis, sickle cell disease

Total parenteral nutrition, especially long term intravenous feeding in premature babies

Cystic fibrosis

Bowel resection and terminal ileum anomalies

Malabsorption

Hepatitis

Any severe illness associated with prolonged fasting. These gallstones may resolve on recovery from the underlying illness

Congenital biliary anomalies

Frusemide therapy

2.24 ARTEFACTS MIMICKING GALLSTONES

Partial volume – usually due to impression by the duodenum

Refraction shadows from folds in the gallbladder neck

Respiratory motion artefact – little problem with real time scanners

Shadows arising directly anterior or posterior to the gallbladder e.g. rib

Inspissated bile sludge – commonly seen in ill patients

Junctional mucosal fold

Any cause of intraluminal filling defect

2.25 FILLING DEFECTS IN THE GALLBLADDER

Gallstones
Sludge/debris
Pus
Blood clot
Artefacts e.g. partial volume
Mucosal folds e.g. junctional fold at the
  junction of the gallbladder body and neck
Cholesterol plaques
Cholesterosis – strawberry gallbladder
  (multiple fixed mural plaques)
Adenoma
Papilloma
Pseudomass – due to impression by
  duodenum
Adenomyomatosis – Rokitansky–Aschoff
  sinuses, may only be visible after
  gallbladder contraction, fundal filling defect,
  local or diffuse stricture
Mucosal hypertrophy/hyperplasia
Inflammatory polyp
Epithelial cyst
Mucus retention cyst
Carcinoma – diagnosis is difficult, gallbladder
  is usually non-functioning and contains
  stones
Metastasis
Carcinoid tumour
Worms and parasites
Ectopic pancreatic tissue
Ectopic gastric tissue
Parasitic granuloma
Varices

Tortuous artery/aneurysm
Food – entero-biliary fistula

2.26 NON-SHADOWING MOBILE INTRALUMINAL GALLBLADDER DEFECTS

Calculi
Bile sludge
Pseudosludge – artefact due to partial volume
  effect
Blood
Pus
Food/faeces
Fibrinous debris/desquamated mucosa
Ascaris lumbricoides
Fasciola hepatica
Clonorchis sinensis

2.27 LOW LEVEL ECHOES IN THE GALLBLADDER

Concentration of bile in fasting patients may
  give rise to sludge formation. This is
  slightly echogenic but does not shadow and
  may form a fluid/sludge level.
Cholesterol crystals – small but very
  echogenic
Multiple small stones
Pus
Abnormal mucus
Parasites/worms

In the majority of patients bile sludge of low echogenicity is a transient phenomenon which passes as the patient's general health improves. Patients with fine echogenic gravel within the gallbladder are found to have gallstones which were obscured by the gravel in 60 % of cases. The remaining 40 % of cases usually show evidence at operation of acute or chronic cholecystitis.

2.28 STRUCTURES MIMICKING THE GALLBLADDER

Duodenal cap and fluid filled bowel loops
Hepatic cysts
Omental cysts
Ligamentum teres abscess
Choledochal cysts
Solitary renal cysts
Dilated cystic duct remnant after
  cholecystectomy

2.29 NON-VISUALIZATION OF THE GALLBLADDER

Post-prandial gallbladder contraction
Chronic cholecystitis
Gallbladder obscured by gas. (Gallbladder
  obscured by or mistaken for a bowel loop)
Ectopic gallbladder e.g. intrahepatic/
  suprahepatic
Post cholecystectomy
Congenital absence (0.03 % of patients)
Porcelain gallbladder
Gangrenous cholecystitis
Emphysematous cholecystitis
Carcinoma of the gallbladder
Metastases invading the gallbladder/
  gallbladder bed
Acute hepatic dysfunction e.g. hepatitis
Technical factors e.g. obesity, very thin patient
  with a superficial gallbladder

2.30 INCREASED GALLBLADDER WALL THICKNESS

Anterior gallbladder wall thickness 3 mm or
more
Fasting (3.5 % of fasting patients show
transient gallbladder wall thickening)
Artefactual – oblique sections, poor distension
(post prandial)
Acute cholecystitis
Chronic cholecystitis
Hypoproteinaemia/hypoalbuminaemia
Cirrhosis
Right heart failure/congestive cardiac failure
Renal failure
Hepatitis
Acute pancreatitis
Ascites. Increased gallbladder wall thickness
may be artefactual
Focal obstruction to gallbladder lymphatic
drainage e.g. nodes at the porta hepatis
Gallbladder torsion
Systemic venous hypertension
Adenomyomatosis
Fat/pathology adjacent to the gallbladder in
the gallbladder fossa
Portal hypertension
Myeloma
AIDS
Xanthogranulomatous cholecystitis
Carcinoma of the gallbladder
Infectious mononucleosus
Acute alcohol abuse

2.30.1 Acute cholecystitis

Acute inflammation of the gallbladder is usually bacterial in origin but may be sterile. The majority of cases are associated with the presence of gallstones, the inflammatory episode being precipitated by impaction of a gallstone in the cystic duct. Distension of the gallbladder by mucus causes venous congestion and eventually leads to arterial embarrassment and ischaemia. If the obstructed gallbladder does not become infected then distension by mucus leads to mucocoele formation. Infection in these cases causes acute cholecystitis. If medical treatment is given early in an attack 95 % of cases resolve but at least 50 % will have further attacks.

A *Sonographic features of acute cholecystitis*

Calculi in gallbladder, Hartmann's pouch or cystic duct. The latter may be hard to detect

Anterior gallbladder wall greater than 3 mm thick

Positive ultrasonic Murphy's sign

Pericholecystic fluid collection in severe cases. A sign of actual or impending perforation

Echopoor halo in or around the gallbladder wall

Non-visualization of the gallbladder in a truly fasting patient is strong evidence of gallbladder disease

Acalculous cholecystitis. Five per cent of cases are not associated with gallstones

Gallbladder distension. Ninety-three per cent of patients with a gallbladder volume over 70 ml have acute cholecystitis

Increased periportal echogenicity. This is presumably due to a local inflammatory infiltrate

Loss of definition of gallbladder margins

Cystic duct obstruction is present in over 95 % of cases of acute cholecystitis. This may be demonstrated by HIDA isotope scanning. In fasting patients HIDA excreted in the bile outlines the gallbladder. Lack of gallbladder visualization is presumptive evidence of cystic duct obstruction and is 94–100 % accurate as a marker for acute cholecystitis.

2.30.2 False positive results at HIDA scan

i.e. lack of gallbladder visualization:

> Prolonged fasting
> Total parenteral nutrition
> Inadequate fasting
> Acute pancreatitis
> Acute alcoholic hepatitis
> Cirrhosis
> Gallbladder hydrops

2.30.3 Chronic cholecystitis

The sonographic diagnosis of chronic cholecystitis is less reliable than acute cholecystitis. Lack of gallbladder visualization in a truly fasting patient is virtually diagnostic of gallbladder disease but many cases simply show evidence of gallstones with or without gallbladder wall thickening. As gallstones are common these findings do not necessarily indicate that they are the cause for the patient's symptoms. ERCP may also be unhelpful as an abnormal gallbladder may distend during a contrast injection yet it may not distend under physiological conditions. The most reliable sign of chronic cholecystitis is a shrunken gallbladder containing gallstones but care must be taken not to mistake a bowel loop for a contracted gallbladder in a non-fasting patient.

2.30.4 Acalculous cholecystitis

Infection may occur secondary to bile stasis without the presence of gallstones. Bile stasis usually occurs due to other intercurrent illness particularly with fever and dehydration. Up to 30 % are jaundiced but as the cystic duct is not obstructed gallbladder distension is less marked than in cases associated with gallstones. Over 50 % of cases of cholecystitis in children occur in the absence of stones but the association with gallstones rises with age.

2.31 CAUSES OF PERI-CHOLECYSTIC FLUID

Acute cholecystitis
Pericholecystic abscess
Ascites
Pancreatitis
Peptic ulcer with or without perforation
Liver abscess
Peritonitis
Ligamentum teres abscess
Ruptured hepatic adenoma
Ruptured ectopic gestation
AIDS

2.31.1 Gallbladder hydrops

Tense gallbladder distension is uncommon in the absence of gallstones, inflammation, lymphadenopathy at the porta hepatis or congenital malformation. The majority of cases occur in children and may follow an acute febrile illness or gastroenteritis. Sonographically the appearances may be indistinguishable from mucocoele of the gallbladder though the latter is usually larger and associated with cystic duct obstruction by stones. Lack of gallbladder drainage may be confirmed by pre- and post-prandial examinations and may be due to transient cystic duct obstruction by sludge or pressure from adjacent lymph nodes.

2.31.2 Emphysematous cholecystitis

Infection with gas forming organisms may give rise to gas in the gallbladder lumen or wall. When gas is prominent the gallbladder may be mistaken for a bowel loop due to the increased echogenicity and shadowing. This rare form of cholecystitis usually affects diabetics or debilitated patients.

A Desquamative cholecystitis

Rarely cholecystitis results in a desquamative process in the gallbladder wall. This gives rise to a bizarre multiseptate appearance.

2.31.3 Carcinoma of the gallbladder

Carcinoma of the gallbladder is not uncommon accounting for up to 3 % of primary malignancies. It is the commonest biliary malignancy and usually occurs in the elderly. Gallbladder carcinoma is commoner in females than males and 73–98 % of cases are associated with gallstones. Twenty-five to sixty-one per cent of cases of porcelain gallbladder are complicated by carcinoma. The carcinoma may be infiltrating causing diffuse thickening and induration of the gallbladder wall or fungating resulting in a mass which fills the gallbladder lumen and invades the wall. Appearances may be indistinguishable from chronic cholecystitis and many cases are only diagnosed at surgery. By this time tumour may have invaded the liver, CBD or lymph nodes and average survival from the time of diagnosis is only five months.

A Sonographic findings

Gallstones within a mass is strongly suspicious of carcinoma of the gallbladder

Localized/diffuse gallbladder wall thickening

Polypoid intraluminal mass

Diffusely echogenic mass

Extensive tumour spread causing obstructive jaundice

Low echogenicity mass extending into porta and liver

Spread from carcinoma of the gallbladder may cause lymphadenopathy in the region of the head of pancreas. This may obstruct the CBD and mimic carcinoma of the head of pancreas. Up to 25 % of cases show calcification in the gallbladder wall or typical appearances of a porcelain gallbladder.

2.31.4 Porcelain gallbladder

A porcelain gallbladder shows diffuse wall calcification seen as a curvilinear densely reflective area with distal acoustic shadowing. It is a rare condition usually associated with chronic inflammation. There is an increased risk of gallbladder carcinoma which complicates 25–61 % of cases however porcelain gallbladder is a rare condition thus the majority of cases of gallbladder carcinoma are not associated with it. The main differential diagnoses for porcelain gallbladder includes:

Bowel loops
Chronic cholecystitis
Cholelithiasis
Emphysematous cholecystitis

2.32 MULTISEPTATE GALLBLADDER

Appearance of normal gallbladder folded over
Congenital multiseptate gallbladder with fine
    nonshadowing septations
Desquamated gallbladder mucosa.
    Hyperplastic cholecystitis. An unusual
    finding in acute cholecystitis giving multiple
    linear nonshadowing echoes in the
    gallbladder lumen in a haphazard
    arrangement
Polypoid cholesterolosis. Non-shadowing
    mural and intraluminal densities which do
    not bridge the lumen
Adenomyomatosis – Rokitansky–Aschoff
    sinuses. These are in the wall and are
    usually quite small. Unless gross they will
    not be confused with a multiseptate
    gallbladder

2.33 HYPERECHOIC FOCI IN THE GALLBLADDER WALL

Cholesterol plaques
Rokitansky–Aschoff sinuses containing stones
   or sludge
Intramural gas bubbles in emphysematous
   cholecystitis
Small adherent stones
Small polyps
Intramural microabscesses

2.34 CHOLECYSTOMEGALY

antero–posterior diameter greater than 4 cm
   Cystic duct obstruction
   Biliary stasis e.g. Prolonged fasting,
      Post surgery,
      IV feeding,
      Post vagotomy stasis,
      Diabetes mellitus
   Hydropic gallbladder – Febrile illness in
      children
      Hepatitis
      Scarlet fever
      Gastroenteritis
      Leptospirosis
      Mucocutaneous lymphnode syndrome,
      (Kawasaki's syndrome)
   Mucocoele of the gallbladder
   AIDS

2.34.1 The pancreas

The pancreas is a 15–20 cm long retroperitoneal organ
with a lobulated outline. It lies on the posterior

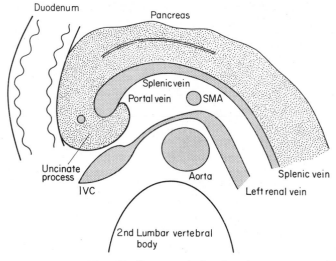

Fig. 12. Pancreatic landmarks.

abdominal wall with its head in the 'c' of the duodenal loop. The body and tail of the gland extend obliquely to the left and the tail lies in the lienorenal ligament. The head of pancreas has an uncinate process which extends postero-inferiorly around the superior mesenteric vein. The gland has no true capsule and may be infiltrated by retroperitoneal fat in obese patients. This may make it difficult to define the pancreatic borders.

A Sonographic landmarks

The head of pancreas lies in the curve of the duodenal loop with the IVC, right renal vessels and CBD lying posteriorly. The neck of pancreas is marked by the union of splenic and superior mesenteric veins posteriorly and the pylorus and gastroduodenal artery anteriorly. The lesser sac is anterior to the body of pancreas and the splenic vein lies on the postero-superior surface. The tail of pancreas is related to the left kidney, adrenal and spleen. (See Fig. 12.)

The retroperitoneum is best examined in the morning as it is easily obscured by overlying bowel gas. The majority of gas within the bowel is swallowed air and this is at a minimum when the patient awakes. When the stomach is empty the pancreas may be visualized by scanning directly through the pylorus either on inspiration or with the stomach pushed out (to displace bowels without overinflating the lungs). The tail of pancreas may be examined through the spleen and left kidney. The gland should demonstrate homogenous echogenicity which is more echogenic than the adjacent liver in 52 % of patients and of equal echogenicity in 48 %. In children the gland is less echogenic than in adults and is relatively larger. The main pancreatic duct can be visualized in up to 85 % of patients depending upon the quality of the scanner. It is seen as a hypoechoic tube around 1.3 mm in diameter though a collapsed duct may have the appearance of a fine echogenic line. The normal pancreatic duct is usually less than 2 mm in diameter though normal ducts of up to 3 mm have been reported in the pancreatic head.

DUCT DIMENSIONS –

Average normal duct diameter 1.3 ± 0.3 mm
Average duct with gallstones 1.4 mm
Acute pancreatitis 2.9 ± 1.1 mm
Resolving pancreatitis 1.7 ± 0.5 mm

The main duct calibre increases with age. Average pancreatic thickness (AP diameter)

Head 2.5–3.5 cm
Body 1.75–2.5 cm
Tail 1.5–3.5 cm

The gland size is very variable depending upon the age and distribution of the population studied hence the variation in the results shown above. Generally the gland decreases in size with age and becomes more echogenic. As with any organ actual measurements serve only as a guide in gland assessment and the overall impression of gland configuration and appearance is often more important. This can only be achieved with experience and over-reliance on measurements in diagnosis will lead to errors.

2.34.2 Acute pancreatitis

Pancreatitis is a relatively common clinical condition with a high morbidity and a significant mortality. The diagnosis is usually made from the clinical history, physical examination and results of serum biochemistry but presentation may be atypical and should be considered as a possible diagnosis in any case of abdominal pain. Up to 80 % of cases are secondary to other disease and sonography is valuable in the assessment of underlying disorders and complications.

A Aetiology

Any pancreatic disease e.g. annular pancreas, pancreas divisum (up to 50 % have episodes of pancreatitis. This is due to failure of fusion of the pancreatic ducts of Wirsung and Santorini and affects 5–11 % of the population.)

Alcohol excess   Gallstones
Peptic ulceration   ERCP

Abdominal operation
Autoimmune disease
Hyperlipidaemia
Hypercalcaemia
Viral infections
Ascariasis
Hereditary

Trauma e.g. biopsy
Congenital/acquired
   pancreatic disease
Hyperparathyroidism
Post renal transplant
   dialysis
Drugs/chemotherapy
   e.g. isoniazid
      rifampicin
      tetracycline
oral contraceptives
   phenformin
   steroids

B Sonographic features

The pancreas may appear normal particularly in
   mild or early cases
Oedema and swelling of the gland may cause enlargement with reduction in parenchymal echogenicity
Echopattern may become heterogenous
The pancreatic duct may be dilated
Adjacent soft tissues may be thickened and/or
   oedematous
Fluid collections occur either due to fluid exudation
   or tissue necrosis. These collections may lie within
   the gland or anteriorly in the lesser sac forming
   pseudocysts. Spread of fluid around the peritoneal
   cavity may result in pancreatic ascites. Secondary
   infection of the inflamed gland or fluid collections
   may give rise to abscess formation and the necrotic
   gland may haemorrhage
Any or all of these changes may occur. They may
   be generalized or focal affecting only part of the
   gland.

2.34.3 Chronic pancreatitis

Recurrent or persistent attacks of pancreatitis lead to irreversible damage. This is particularly likely when the cause of the initial attack persists. Thirty to sixty-five per cent of cases are associated with pancreatic calcification on the plain abdominal radiograph. A rare form of hereditary pancreatitis is associated with pancreatic calcification which may be very prominent, but pancreatic calcification may also occur in any case of chronic pancreatitis including those due to hyperparathyroidism, cystic fibrosis, pancreatic malignancy and kwashiorkor.

A *Sonographic features*

The gland may appear normal even in the presence of advanced disease

In the early stages the gland is enlarged and hypoechoic with duct dilatation

The gland becomes heterogenous with areas of increased echogenicity and focal or diffuse enlargement

Pseudocysts may occur

Focal hypoechoic inflammatory masses may mimic pancreatic neoplasia

Calculi and calcification within the gland give rise to densely echogenic foci which may shadow

The pancreatic and common bile ducts may be dilated

In the late stages of disease the gland becomes atrophic, fibrosed and shrinks. This results in a small echogenic gland with a heterogenous echopattern. The pancreatic duct may remain dilated with a beaded appearance due to multiple stenoses.

2.34.4 Pancreatic pseudocyst

Fluid collections occur in up to 50 % of cases of acute pancreatitis. Pseudocysts are usually seen as anechoic fluid filled spaces but they may show internal echoes if they contain necrotic tissue or clot. Small fluid collections are often transient and collections less than 5 cm in diameter may be treated conservatively. They may dissect tissue planes and thus can present at a distance from the pancreas. They have even been reported in the mediastinum and scrotum. Without treatment some collections may become massive distending the lesser sac or filling the abdomen.

A False positive results

Gallbladder distension
Fluid filled bowel loop
Choledochal cyst
Cystic pancreatic tumour

Aspiration of a pseudocyst increases the risk of infection and should only be carried out when clearly indicated. Surgical drainage requires organization of the pseudocyst wall so that it can hold sutures. Percutaneous drainage may also be performed under ultrasound control, the drain may be inserted through the stomach in a manner similar to marsupialization performed at surgery.

B Cystic fibrosis

Cystic fibrosis causes a pronounced increase in pancreatic echogenicity which is independent of age. Small cysts occur particularly in the pancreatic tail and the gland atrophies resulting in a decreased anteroposterior diameter. Sonography is frequently used to assess changes in gland morphology but sonographic appearances do not correlate well with pancreatic function. Sonography of the pancreas is usually combined with evaluation of the liver, gallbladder, common bile duct, portal venous system and spleen and is more valuable in the assessment of the onset of liver disease with portal hypertension.

C Pancreatic carcinoma

Though pancreatic carcinoma is a classic cause of progressive painless jaundice the commonest presenting symptoms are pain and weight loss. If a mass is identified then ultrasonography may allow guided biopsy. Without biopsy the false positive rate of diagnosis of pancreatic carcinoma is 25 % owing to the frequency of inflammatory masses of identical echopattern. There has been a four-fold rise in the incidence of pancreatic carcinoma over the last 40 years and risk factors include cigarette smoking, asbestos exposure and possibly coffee drinking.

The commonest sonographic appearance of carcinoma of the pancreas is a hypoechoic mass with a heterogenous echopattern. The mass may be visible before the gland is enlarged but identical appearances may occur in pancreatitis. Carcinoma of the pancreas may obstruct the pancreatic duct causing pancreatitis and thus the two conditions may coexist making diagnosis difficult. Seventy per cent of carcinomas occur in the pancreatic head and less than 10 % occur in the tail. Ultrasonography is an accurate screening method for assessment of the pancreatic head and body but visualization of the pancreatic tail is less reliable. Prone and prone-oblique scans through the left renal bed may aid visualization of the pancreatic tail. Carcinoma of the pancreatic tail usually presents at a late stage of disease and metastases are usually present at the time of diagnosis.

CAUSES OF HYPOECHOIC PANCREATIC MASSES –

Carcinoma
Focal pancreatitis/inflammatory masses
Lymphoma
Metastases

SONOGRAPHIC SIGNS OF PANCREATIC CARCINOMA –

Focal or diffuse mass

Usually greater than 2 cm diameter at diagnosis

Mass usually well defined and smooth in outline

Tumours in the body and tail are usually seen as masses that cause changes in the gland shape. Tumours in the gland head begin as focal masses but often cause diffuse enlargement

± pancreatic duct dilatation and pancreatitis. (Pancreatic duct is dilated in up to 97 % of cases of pancreatic carcinoma. The duct diameter should not normally exceed 2 mm Duct dilatation also occurs in pancreatitis but tends to be more irregular than in cases of carcinoma.) (Pancreatitis may give rise to an inflammatory mass which obscures the underlying tumour.)

± CBD dilatation. Occurs in 80–90 % of cases of pancreatic head carcinoma

The majority are hypoechoic but 3 % are echogenic. Once inflammatory changes occur the echopattern may become heterogenous.

With small tumours dilatation of the pancreatic duct may be the only sonographic abnormality. The presence of pancreatic calcification or intraduct calculi makes chronic pancreatitis more likely but does not exclude pancreatic carcinoma.

Forty-seven per cent of cases are associated with hepatic metastases at the time of diagnosis. These may be echopoor or echogenic.

D Masses adjacent to the pancreas may be mistaken for pancreatic masses

e.g.

Retroperitoneal veins/varices
Retroperitoneal masses
Lymphatic masses/nodes
Renal tumours
Arterial aneurysms

2.34.5 Cystic pancreatic neoplasms

Cystadenoma of pancreas. These uncommon tumours account for 10 % of benign pancreatic tumours. They may be microcystic or macrocystic. The latter are usually 2 cm or more in diameter and may be premalignant. They tend to occur in the head of pancreas, may show calcification and are found in women more frequently than men.

Cystadenocarcinoma of pancreas. This rare tumour is the malignant counterpart of macrocystic adenoma of pancreas. It is seen as a solid tumour with cystic elements. Most cases occur in women accounting for 1 % of malignant pancreatic tumours. The tumour forms a well encapsulated and lobulated mass which exhibits slow growth and metastasizes late giving a relatively good prognosis.

2.34.6 Islet cell tumours

These slowly progressive tumours are of low grade malignancy with an overall five-year survival of 44 %. Sixty per cent are insulinomas, 18 % secrete gastrin and 15 % are non-functioning. Functioning and non-functioning islet cell tumours are usually small. In the Zollinger Ellison syndrome only 42 % of tumours are visible sonographically whilst only 30 % of non-functioning islet cell tumours can be identified by ultrasound. In cases of non-functioning tumours angiography is usually more rewarding. When visible islet cell tumours are usually seen as small hypoechoic masses.

2.34.7 Pancreatic sarcoma

Pancreatic sarcoma is seen as a relatively sonolucent mass which may be mistaken for a pseudocyst.

2.34.8 Pancreatic lymphoma

Pancreatic lymphoma gives rise to a large mass which is usually homogenous and sonolucent but may appear complex. There may be lymphadenopathy in the adjacent para-aortic and caval areas.

2.34.9 Pancreatic metastases

Whilst the pancreas is not a particularly common site for metastatic disease, metastases may occur particularly from melanoma, ovary, lung, breast, prostate, hepatoma, hypernephroma and sarcomas. These are usually seen as hypoechoic masses indistinguishable from primary pancreatic tumours.

2.34.10 Lipomatous pseudohypertrophy of the pancreas

This rare condition is associated with diabetes mellitus, obesity, chronic pancreatitis and alcoholic liver disease. There is massive replacement of the pancreas with adipose tissue causing pancreatic enlargement with a heterogenous echopattern.

2.34.11 Pancreatic cysts

Unlike the liver and kidneys, asymptomatic pancreatic cysts are uncommon. Pancreatic cysts may occur in combination with polycystic disease elsewhere, particularly those with an autosomal dominant inheritance. Acquired cysts include retention cysts, hydatid infection, cystic neoplasms and pseudocysts.

2.35 CYSTIC MASS LESIONS OF THE PANCREAS

Pseudocyst/fluid collection
Focal pancreatitis. (May be mistaken for a
 fluid collection)
Abscess
Dilated distal CBD
Congenital cysts
Acquired cysts
Haematoma
Hydatid cyst
Microcystic adenomas
Mucinous cystic tumours
Necrotic primary or secondary tumour e.g.
 pancreatic carcinoma, leiomyosarcoma
Cystic pancreatic tumour
Lymphoma. (May appear anechoic and mimic
 a fluid collection)

2.35.1 The spleen

In the young adult the spleen is approximately $3 \times 8 \times 13$ cm and weighs 200–300 g but size is very variable and may change in a short space of time in response to infection and other stresses. It is larger in relation to total size in children and decreases in size in middle and old age. Accessory splenic tissue or splenuncule is found in 20–30 % of post-mortems. These accessory spleens are usually found around the splenic hilum. They are not usually visible sonographically except when the spleen is enlarged but may simulate pancreatic tail masses. The splenic parenchyma is usually more echogenic than adjacent kidney and similar in appearance to the liver.

2.35.2 Splenomegaly

The size and shape of the spleen are very variable, some being long and thin whilst others are short and thick. This variation, together with the natural tendency of splenic size to vary during infective episodes, makes assessment of minor changes in size very subjective. Despite this splenomegaly is usually demonstrable sonographically before it is clinically evident. The enlarged spleen may extend inferiorly over the left kidney improving renal visualization. When very large the spleen may extend into the left iliac fossa. Any spleen over 13 cm long should be considered enlarged particularly if it also shows increased antero-posterior diameter.

2.35.3 Splenic trauma

The spleen is prone to injury by blunt abdominal trauma. Ultrasonography is valuable both for the demonstration of splenic haematomas and lacerations and also for the examination of other organs such as liver and kidneys which may also be damaged. Small volumes of intraperitoneal fluid may also be demonstrated and in the context of abdominal trauma this may be assumed to be due to the presence of blood.

2.35.4 Splenic haematoma

Splenic haematomas are initially seen as anechoic collections which may become echogenic as the blood clots. Later liquefaction of the haematoma may give a complex or cystic appearance. Subcapsular collections conform closely to the splenic shape. These may rupture some time after the trauma causing late but severe haemorrhage.

2.35.5 Splenic lacerations

Splenic lacerations are reliably demonstrated provided the spleen can be adequately visualized. This is often difficult after trauma as the patient is usually acutely tender in the area of interest. Lacerations are seen as anechoic defects in the splenic margin and parenchyma. This is due to the presence of blood within the laceration. As the blood clots the laceration may appear echogenic.

2.35.6 Splenectomy

The spleen is a very vascular organ and laceration may cause torrential haemorrhage. Laceration may occur with minimal trauma particularly if the spleen is diseased e.g. by infectious mononucleosis. Splenectomy is avoided if at all possible particularly in children as there is a very high post-splenectomy rate of infection. (After splenectomy children have a 60 times average risk of death from sepsis such as pneumonia and meningitis.) Despite this, splenectomy may be necessary to prevent fatal haemorrhage and the sonographer should recognize the progressive signs of splenic haemorrhage ranging from the early subcapsular haematoma or laceration to the build up of peritoneal fluid due to persistent bleeding. After splenectomy fluid collections may occur in the left upper quadrant or bowel loops may fall into the splenic bed mimicking post operative abscess.

2.35.7 Splenic abscess

Despite the vascular nature of the spleen and the frequency of septicaemia splenic abscesses are uncommon.

A Aetiology

75 % are due to haematological spread of infection, particularly in IV drug abuse

15 % follow trauma with haematological spread to a haematoma

10 % are due to spread of infection from adjacent organs such as colon or subphrenic abscess

Splenic abscess is seen as an anechoic or hypoechoic focus which is usually ill-defined but can be well defined with a recognizable wall. There may be internal debris or even gas bubbles giving rise to highly echogenic foci.

The diagnosis of splenic abscess is usually suggested by the clinical history, the main differential diagnosis in these circumstances being a splenic haematoma or haemorrhagic infarct.

2.35.8 Splenic infarction

Splenic infarction is not uncommon and is usually the result of another disease process such as sickle cell anaemia, leukaemia, subacute bacterial endocarditis, systemic lupus erythematosus etc. The spleen is often acutely painful and this may make sonography difficult. Initially the spleen appears normal but a wedge-shaped hypoechoic area forms representing the infarct. This later becomes echogenic and may atrophy leaving a small echogenic scar. Haemorrhage into the infarct will change its appearance making it anechoic, hypoechoic or complex depending upon the stage of haemorrhage. Repeated infarcts may lead to auto-splenectomy with a small spleen with multiple echogenic nodules representing old infarcts.

2.35.9 Splenic cysts

Cysts may be true congenital cysts with an epithelial lining or acquired cysts due to previous infection or trauma. Congenital cysts have the same appearance as simple cysts elsewhere in the body. They are well defined anechoic spaces with no demonstrable wall or capsule. There is distal acoustic enhancement and unless the cyst has been complicated by infection or haemorrhage there are no internal echoes. Simple cysts are far less common in the spleen than renal or hepatic cysts but they are by no means rare. Haematomas may form cysts as they liquefy and often the patient cannot clearly recall the episode of trauma responsible. Hydatid cysts are the most important infective cysts in the spleen, their appearance is that of hydatid disease in the liver. Both hydatid cysts and haematomas may calcify.

A Splenic cysts – differential diagnosis

> Parasitic e.g. hydatid
> Primary cysts with a true cellular lining
>   e.g. endothelial lining   – haemangioma
>   – lymphangioma
>   epithelial lining   – dermoid
>   – epidermoid
>   – transitional cell lined
> Secondary cysts without a true cellular lining
>   e.g. traumatic cysts

2.35.10 Splenic malignancy

The spleen may be primarily involved in a malignant process such as lymphoma or uncommonly it may be the site of metastatic disease. Focal splenic involvement in lymphoma is uncommon and is easily missed. When visible this is seen as hypoechoic or anechoic foci. With diffuse splenic involvement lymphoma and leukaemia may simply give rise to splenomegaly which may be indistinguishable from other causes of splenic enlargement. In addition splenomegaly may occur as a reactive process to disease elsewhere and does not always indicate splenic involvement. Furthermore the great variation in splenic size from person to person makes the diagnosis of lesser degrees of splenic enlargement unreliable though ultrasonography remains a more sensitive indicator of splenomegaly than palpation.

Though the spleen is very vascular it is an uncommon site for metastases. Metastatic colonic carcinoma in the spleen has been reported to have an echogenic appearance and metastatic melanoma has been reported to give both echogenic and hypoechoic appearances.

2.35.11 Granulomatous splenic infections

The most commonly encountered granulomatous splenic infections are tuberculosis and histoplasmosis. Infection occurs secondary to haematogenous spread from disease elsewhere and if symptoms occur they are usually due to generalized disease and not local splenic involvement. Miliary tuberculosis may give rise to a generally bright echopattern but this appearance is non-specific and may also occur in other inflammatory states and untreated malignancy. Healed granulomas calcify giving rise to multiple echogenic foci which may be visible on a plain abdominal radiograph.

2.36 SPLENIC CALCIFICATION

Cyst wall calcification
Old abscess
Calcified granuloma
Healed infarct
Old haematoma
Splenic artery aneurysm at the splenic hilum
Phleboliths
Haemangioma
Brucellosis

2.37 MULTIFOCAL HYPOECHOIC SPLENIC MASSES

Splenic lymphangiomatosis
Lymphoma
Infarction. Lesions usually of different ages
   and therefore of varying appearances
Septic emboli – multiple small abscesses
Metastases e.g. melanoma, breast, ovary,
   lung, hepatoma, endometrial carcinoma,
   stomach
Splenic cysts e.g. simple, epidermoid, hydatid
Abscesses

2.38 FLUID FILLED LEFT UPPER QUADRANT MASS

Stomach
Left renal cyst
Necrotic renal tumour
Left adrenal cyst
Necrotic left adrenal tumour
Pancreatic pseudocyst
Pancreatic cystadenoma/cystadenocarcinoma
Abscess
Haematoma
Splenic cyst
Hepatic cyst in left lobe of liver
Loculated ascites
Splenic artery aneurysm
Hydronephrosis
Pseudo-perisplenic fluid – anechoic soft tissue
   mistaken for fluid e.g. lymphoma

2.39 SPLENOMEGALY WITH A NORMAL ECHOPATTERN

Infection (non-specific reaction to distant focal or general infection)
Hepatocellular disease
Sickle cell disease (later spleen is small due to infarcts)
Hereditary spherocytosis
Leukaemia
Haemolysis
Chronic anaemia
Still's disease
Felty's syndrome
Wilson's disease
Reticulum cell sarcoma

2.40 SPLENOMEGALY WITH A HYPOECHOIC ECHOPATTERN

Hepatocellular disease
Hodgkin's disease
Myeloma
Non-caseous granulomatous inflammation
Leukaemia

2.41 SOLID HETEROGENOUS SPLENIC MASS LESIONS

Haematoma
Abscess
Infarcts
Angiosarcoma
Haemangioma
Haemangiosarcoma

2.42 ECHOGENIC SPLENIC MASSES

Infarcts
Haematoma
Metastases
Hereditary spherocytosis
Calcification in granulomata

FURTHER READING

Abbitt P L & Teates C D. The sonographic appearance of extramedullary haematopoiesis in the liver. *J. Clin. Ult.* (1989) **17**: 280–282.

Abul-Khair M H *et al*. Ultrasonography of amoebic liver abscesses. *Ann. Surg.* (1981) **193** (2): 221–226.

Alibone G W *et al*. Sonographic features of carcinoma of the gall bladder. *Gastrointest. Radiol.* (1981) **6**: 169–173.

Alpern M A *et al*. Chronic pancreatitis: ultrasonic features. *Radiology* (1985) **155**: 215–219.

Andrew W K & Glynthomas R. Hydatid cyst of the pancreatic tail. *South Af. Med. J.* (1981) **7**: 235–236.

Arger P H *et al*. An analysis of pancreatic sonography in pancreatic disease. *J. Clin. Ult.* (1979) **7**: 91–97.

Barnett E & Morley P. Eds. *Clinical Diagnostic Ultrasound*. Blackwell Scientific Publications (1985).

Barriga P *et al*. An ultrasonographically solid, tumour-like appearance of echinococcal cysts in the liver. *J. Ult. Med.* (1983) **2**: 123–125.

Beinhart C *et al*. Obstruction without dilatation. *J. Am. Med. Assoc.* (1982) **245**: 353–356.

Bellamy P R & Hicks A. Implications for dissolution therapy. *Clin. Rad.* (1988) **39**: 511–512.

Berger L A. Chronic afferent loop obstruction diagnosed by ultrasound. *Brit. J. Rad.* (1980) **53**: 810–812.

Berk R N *et al*. *Radiology of the Gall Bladder and Bile Ducts*. W B Saunders (1983) pp. 515–518.

Berland LL. Focal areas of decreased echogenicity in the liver at the porta hepatis. *J. Ult. Med.* (1986) **5**: 157–159.

Bevan G. Tumours of the gall bladder. *Clin. Gastroent.* (1973) **2**: 175–184.

Bloom R A *et al*. The ultrasound spectrum of emphysematous cholecystitis. *J. Clin. Ult.* (1989) **17**: 251–265.

Bolandi L *et al*. Ultrasonography in the diagnosis of portal hypertension. Diminished response of portal vessels to respiration. *Radiology* (1982) **142**: 167–172.

Bressler E L *et al*. Sonographic parallel channel sign: A reappraisal. *Radiology* (1987) **164**: 343–346.

Brunelle F & Chaumont P. Hepatic tumours in children, ultrasonic differentiation of benign and malignant lesion. *Radiology* (1984) **150**: 695–699.

Bundy A L & Richie W G M. Ultrasonic diagnosis of metastatic melanoma presenting as acute cholecystitis. *J. Clin. Ult.* (1982) **10**: 285–287.

Bryan P J. Appearance of normal pancreatic duct: a study using real-time ultrasound. *J. Clin. Ult.* (1982) **10**: 63–66.

Carroll B A. Gall bladder wall thickening secondary

to focal lymphatic obstruction. *J. Ult. Med.* (1983) **2**: 89–91.

Carroll B A & Oppenheimer D A. Sclerosing cholangitis: sonographic demonstration of bile duct wall thickening. *Am. J. Roent.* (1982) **139**: 1016–1018.

Carters V̄ *et al.* Papillary adenoma of the gall bladder, ultrasonic demonstration. *J. Clin. Ult.* (1978) **6**: 433–435.

Chau E M T *et al.* Prominent periportal echogenicity, its sonographic evaluation and its significance. *Brit. J. Rad.* (1986) **59**: 543–546.

Coleman B G *et al.* Greyscale sonographic assessment of pancreatitis in children. *Radiology* (1983) **146**: 145–150.

Cosgrove D O & Bark M. Ultrasound in the diagnosis of liver disease. In *Clinical Radiology of the Liver.* Herlinger H ed, Marcel Dekker, New York (1983).

Cotton P B *et al.* Greyscale ultrasonography and endoscopic pancreatography in pancreatic diagnosis. *Radiology* (1980) **134**: 453–459.

Crade M & Taylor K J W. Ultrasound diagnosis of pancreatic pathology. *J. Clin. Gastroent.* (1979) **1**: 171–181.

Crivello M S *et al.* Left lobe of liver mimicking perisplenic collections. *J. Clin. Ult.* (1986) **14**: 697–701.

Crowley S F & Hedvall S E. Cystic duct remnant, sonographic diagnosis. *J. Ult. Med.* (1985) **4**: 261–263.

Dachman A H *et al.* Non parasitic splenic cysts. A report of 52 cases with radiologic pathologic correlation. *Am. J. Roent.* (1986) **147**: 537–542.

Dalla Palma L *et al.* Greyscale Ultrasonography in evaluation of carcinoma of the gall bladder. *Brit. J. Rad.* (1980) **53**: 662–667.

Dewbury K. The features of the Mirizzi syndrome on ultrasound examination. *Brit. J. Rad.* (1979) **52**: 990.

Dewbury K C & Clark B. The accuracy of ultrasound detection of cirrhosis of the liver. *Brit. J. Rad.* (1979) **52**: 945–948.

Didier D *et al*. Hepatic alveolar echinococcosis: correlative ultrasound and CT study. *Radiology* (1985) **154**: 179–186.

Do Carmo M *et al*. Natural history study of gall bladder cancer. *Cancer* (1978) **42**: 330–335.

Doust B D. Ultrasonic examination of the pancreas. *Rad. Clin. North Am.* (1975) **13**: 467–478.

Doust B D & Pearce J D. Greyscale ultrasonic properties of the normal and inflamed pancreas. *Radiology* (1976) **120**: 653–657.

Doust B D *et al*. Ultrasonic distinction of abscesses from other intra-abdominal fluid collections. *Radiology* (1977) **125**: 213–218.

Duddy M J & Calder C J. Cystic haemangioma of the spleen: findings on ultrasound and CT. *Brit. J. Rad.* (1989) **62** (734): 180–182.

Durrell C A *et al*. Gall bladder ultrasonography in clinical context. *Seminars Ultrason., CT & MR* (1984) **5** (4).

El Shafic M & Meeh C L. Transient gall bladder distension in sick premature infants: the value of ultrasonography and radionuclide scintigraphy. *Paed. Rad.* (1986) **16**: 468–471.

Elyaderoi M K & Gabriele O F. Cholecystosonography in the detection of acute cholecystitis: the halo sign: a significant sonographic finding. *South. Med. J.* (1983) **76**: 174–180.

Engelhart G & Blauenstein V M. Ultrasound in the

diagnosis of malignant pancreatic tumours. *Gut* (1970) **11**: 443–449.

Enterline D S *et al*. Cyst of falciform ligament of liver. *Am. J. Roent.* (1984) **142**: 327–328.

Fahim R B *et al*. Carcinoma of the gall bladder, a study of its modes and spread. *Ann. Surg.* (1962) **156**: 114–129.

Federle M P *et al*. Cystic hepatic neoplasms: complementary roles of CT and sonography. *Am. J. Roent.* (1981) **136**: 345–348.

Federle M P *et al*. Recurrent pyogenic cholangitis in Asian immigrants. *Radiology* (1982) **143**: 151–156.

Ferin P & Lerner R. Contracted gall bladder, a finding in hepatic dysfunction. *Radiology* (1985) **154**: 769–770.

Ferrucci J T T R. Radiology of the pancreas. *Rad. Clin. North Am.* (1976) **14**: 543–561.

Filly R A & London S S. The normal pancreas: acoustical characteristics and frequency imaging. *J. Clin. Ult.* (1979) **7**: 121–124.

Fiske C E & Filly R A. Pseudosludge. *Radiology* (1982) **144**: 631–632.

Fiske C E *et al*. Ultrasonic evidence of gall bladder wall thickening in association with hypoalbuminaemia. *Radiology* (1980) **135**: 713–716.

Fontana G *et al*. On evaluation of echography in the diagnoses of pancreatic disease. *Gut* (1976) **17**: 228–234.

Forest E M *et al*. Biliary cystadenomas: sonographic and pathologic correlations. *Am. J. Roent.* (1980) **135**(4): 723–727.

Foster K J *et al*. The accuracy of ultrasound in the detection of fatty infiltration of the liver. *Brit. J. Rad.* (1980) **53**: 440–442.

Fowler R C & Reid W A. Ultrasound diagnosis of adenomyomatosis of the gall bladder: ultrasonic and pathological correlation. *Clin. Rad.* (1988) **39**: 402–406.

Freeny C P & Lawson T L. *Radiology of the Pancreas.* Springer Verlag (1982).

Frick M P & Feinberg S B. Biliary cystadenomas. *Am. J. Roent.* (1982) **139**: 393–395.

Gharbi H A *et al.* Ultrasound examination of the hydatic liver. *Radiology* (1981) **139**: 459–463.

Gibney R G *et al.* Sonographically detected hepatic haemangioma: absence of change over time. *Am. J. Roent.* (1987) **149**: 953–957.

Giorgio A *et al.* Ultrasound evaluation of uncomplicated and complicated viral hepatitis. *J. Clin. Ult.* (1986) **14**: 675–679.

Giyanoni V L *et al.* Omental cyst mimicking the gall bladder. *J. Clin. Ult.* (1986) **14**: 131–133.

Glazer G M *et al.* Demonstration of portal hypertension: the patent umbilical vein. *Radiology* (1980) **136**: 161–163.

Goneling G A W. Food particles in the gall bladder mimicking cholelithiasis in a patient with cholecystojejunostomy. *J. Clin. Ult.* (1981) **9**: 346–347.

Graif M *et al.* Hyperechoic foci in the gall bladder wall, a sign of microabscess formation or diverticula. *Radiology* (1984) **152**: 781–784.

Greenfield R A *et al.* Jaundice, cholelithiasis and a non-dilated CBD. *J. Am. Med. Assoc.* (1978) **240**: 1983–1984.

Gupta R & Woodham C H. Unusual ultrasound appearance of the spleen a case of hereditary spherocytosis. *Brit. J. Rad.* (1986) **59**: 284–285.

Haber K *et al.* Demonstration and dimensional analysis

of the normal pancreas with greyscale echography. *Am. J. Roent.* (1976) **126** (3): 624–628.

Hadidi A. Ultrasonic findings in liver hydatid cysts. *J. Clin. Ult.* (1979) **7**: 365–368.

Hadidi A. Pancreatic duct diameter: sonographic measurements in normal subjects. *J. Clin. Ult.* (1983) **11**: 17–22.

Hadidi A. Sonography of hepatic echinococcal cysts. *Gastrointest. Radiol.* (1982) **7**: 349–354.

Hammond I. Unusual causes of sonographic non-visualisation or non-recognition of the gall bladder: a review. *J. Clin. Ult.* (1988) **16**: 77–85.

Hammond D I & Maclean R S. Gall bladder wall thickening in an elderly woman with infectious mononucleosis. *J. Clin. Ult.* (1987) **15**: 558–560.

Han B K *et al*. Choledochal cyst with bile duct dilatation sonography and 99m TC IDA cholescintigraphy. *Am. J. Roent.* (1981) **136**: 1075–1079.

Hanada K *et al*. Radiologic findings in xanthogranulomatous cholecystitis. *Am. J. Roent.* (1987) **148**: 727–730.

Harbin W *et al*. Non-visualised gall bladder by cholecystosonography. *Am. J. Roent.* (1979) **132**: 727.

Henschke C *et al*. The hyperechogenic liver in children: cause and sonographic appearances. *Am. J. Roent.* (1982) **138**: 841–846.

Hillman B J *et al*. Ultrasonic appearances of the falciform ligament. *Am. J. Roent.* (1979) **132**: 205–206.

Howard R. Acute acalculous cholecystitis. *Am. J. Surg.* (1981) **141**: 194.

Jayonthi V *et al*. Pre-operative and post-operative ultrasound evaluation of the Budd–Chiari syndrome due to coarctation of the inferior vena cava. *Clin. Radiol.* (1988) **39**: 154–158.

Jeasty P *et al.* Mobile intraluminal masses of the gall bladder. *J. Ult. Med.* (1983) **2**: 65–71.

Johnson M L & Mack L A. Ultrasonic evaluation of the pancreas. *Gastrointest. Radiol.* (1978) **3**: 257–266.

Joseph A E A & Dewsbury K C. Ultrasound detection of chronic liver disease (the bright liver). *Brit. J. Rad.* (1979) **52**: 945–948.

Jullner H V *et al.* Thickening of the gall bladder wall in acute hepatitis ultrasound demonstration. *Radiology* (1982) **142**: 465–466.

Jüttner H U *et al.* Ultrasound demonstration of portosystemic collaterals in cirrhosis and portal hypertension. *Radiology* (1982) **142**: 459–463.

Kangarloo H *et al.* Ultrasonographic spectrum of choledochal cysts in childhood. *Paed. Rad.* (1980) **9**: 15.

Kauzlavic D & Passega E. Atypical sonographic findings in splenic infarction. *J. Clin. Ult.* (1986) **14**: 461–462.

Klatskin G. Adenocarcinoma of the hepatic duct at its bifurcation within the porta hepatis. An unusual tumour with distinctive clinical and pathological features. *Am. J. Med.* (1965) **38**: 241–256.

Komaki S & Clark J M. Pancreatic pseudocyst, a review of 17 cases with emphasis on radiological findings. *Am. J. Roent.* (1974) **122**: 385–397.

Koss J C *et al.* Mucocutaneous lymphnode syndrome with hydrops of the gall bladder diagnosed by ultrasound. *J. Clin. Ult.* (1981) **9**: 477–479.

Kuligowska E *et al.* Liver abscess: sonography in diagnosis and treatment. *Am. J. Roent.* (1982) **138**: 253–257.

Laffey P A *et al.* Haemobilia, a cause of false negative ductal dilatation. *J. Clin. Ult.* (1986) **150**: 123–127.

Laing F C & Jeffry R B. The pseudodilated CBD, ultrasonic appearances created by the gall bladder neck. *Radiology* (1980) **135**: 405–407.

Lee J K T *et al*. Pancreatic imaging by ultrasound and computed tomography a general review. *Rad. Clin. North Am.* (1979) **16**: 105–117.

Lee T G *et al*. Ultrasound diagnosis of common bile duct dilatation. *Radiology* (1977) **124**: 793–797.

Lees *et al*. Carcinoma of the bile ducts. *Surg. Gynaecol. Obstet.* (1980) **151**: 193–198.

Leopold G R. Ultrasonography of Jaundice. *Rad. Clin. North Am.* (1979) **XVIII** (1): 127–136.

Leopold G R. Echographic study of the pancreas. *J. Am. Med. Assoc.* (1975) **232**: 287–289.

Leopold G R & Asher W M. *Fundamentals of Abdominal and Pelvic Ultrasonography*. W B Saunders (1975).

Lev-Toaff A S *et al*. Multiseptate gall bladder: incidental diagnosis on sonography. *Am. J. Roent.* (1987) **148**: 1119–1120.

Lewall D B & McCorkell S J. Hepatic echinococcal cysts: sonographic appearances and classification. *Radiology* (1985) **155**: 773–775.

Lewandowski B J & Winsberg F. Gall bladder wall thickness demonstrated by ascites. *Am. J. Roent.* (1981) **137**: 519–521.

Lloyd-Jones W *et al*. Symptomatic non-parasitic cysts of the liver. *Brit. J. Surg.* (1974) **61**: 118–123.

Lorigan J G *et al*. Atrophy with compensatory hypertrophy of the liver with hepatic neoplasms: radiographic findings. *Am. J. Roent.* (1988) **150**: 1291–1295.

Machan L *et al*. Sonographic diagnosis of Klatskin tumours. *Am. J. Roent.* (1986) **147**: 509–512.

Madrazo B L *et al*. Sonographic findings in complicated

peptic ulcer. *Radiology* (1981) **140**: 457–461.

Maffessanti M M *et al*. Sonographic diagnosis in intra-ductal hepatoma. *J. Clin. Ult.* (1982) 397–399.

Malini S & Sabel J. Ultrasonography in obstructive jaundice. *Radiology* (1977) **123**: 429–433.

Marchal *et al*. Caroli Disease: high frequency ultra-sound and pathologic findings. *Radiology* (1986) **158**: 507–511.

Maresca G *et al*. Sonographic patterns of splenic infarction. *J. Clin. Ult.* (1986) **14**: 23–28.

McArdle C R. Ultrasound of the liver metastasis. *J. Clin. Ult.* (1976) **4**: 265–268.

Meyer D G *et al*. Klatskin tumours of the bile ducts, sonographic appearances. *Radiology* (1983) **148**: 803–804.

Miller H J & Greenspan B S. Integrated imaging of hepatic tumours in childhood. *Radiology* (1985) **154**: 91–100.

Miller J M. The ultrasonic appearance of cystic hepato-blastoma. *Radiology* (1981) **138**: 141–143.

Mitchell S E *et al*. The hypoechoic caudate lobe: an ultrasonic pseudolesion. *Radiology* (1982) **144**: 569–572.

Mittelstaedt C A & Partain C L. Ultrasonic – pathologic classification of splenic abnormalities. Greyscale patterns. *Radiology* (1980) **134**: 697–705.

Morrecki *et al*. In: *Neonatal – Perinatal Medicine. Disease of the Foetus and Infant.* C V Mosby ed. Behrman, St Louis (1977).

Murphy F B *et al*. Budd–Chiari syndrome: a review. *Am. J. Roent.* (1986) **147**: 9–15.

Nahman B & Cunningham J J. Sonography of splenic angiosarcoma. *J. Clin. Ult.* (1985) **13**: 354–356.

Newlis N *et al*. Ultrasonic features of pyogenic liver abscess. *Radiology* (1981) **139**: 155–159.

Niccolini D G *et al*. Tumour induced acute pancreatitis. *Gastroenterology* (1976) **71**: 142–145.

Niederau C *et al*. Extrahepatic bile ducts in healthy subjects, in patients with cholelithiasis and post cholecystectomy patients: a prospective ultrasonic study. *J. Clin. Ult.* (1983) **11**: 23–27.

Nyberg D A & Laing F C. Ultrasonic findings in peptic ulcer disease and pancreatitis that simulate primary gall bladder disease. *J. Ult. Med.* (1983) **2**: 303–307.

Okuda K *et al*. Demonstration of growing casts of hepatocellular carcinoma in the portal vein by coeliac angiography, the thread and streaks sign. *Radiology* (1975) **117**: 303–309.

Okuda K *et al*. Clinical aspects of intrahepatic bile duct carcinoma including hilar carcinoma. A study of 57 autopsy proven cases. *Cancer* (1977) **39**: 232–246.

Parulekar S G. Ultrasonic evaluation of the pancreatic duct. *J. Clin. Ult.* (1980) **10**: 63–66.

Patriguin H B *et al*. Sonography of thickened gall bladder wall, causes in children. *Am. J. Roent.* (1983) **141**: 57–60.

Pawar S *et al*. Sonography of splenic abscesses. *Am. J. Roent.* (1982) **138**: 259–262.

Pearl G S & Nassan V H. Cystic lymphangioma of the spleen. *South. Med. J.* (1979) **72**: 667–669.

Peihler J M & Crichlow R W. Primary carcinoma of the gall bladder. *Surg. Gynaecol. Obstet.* (1978) **147**: 929–942.

Phillips G *et al*. Ultrasound patterns of metastatic tumours in the gall bladder. *J. Clin. Ult.* (1982) **10**: 379–383.

Pistoria F & Markowitz S K. Splenic lymphangiomatosis, CT diagnosis. *Am. J. Roent.* (1988) **150**: 121–122.

Power S *et al.* Sonography of splenic abscesses. *Am. J. Roent.* (1982) **138**: 259–262.

Prando A *et al.* Ultrasonic pseudolesions of the liver. *Radiology* (1979) **130**: 403–407.

Price R J *et al.* Sonography of polypoid cholesterosis. *Am. J. Roent.* (1982) **139**: 1197–1198.

Pulpeiro J R *et al.* Primary hepatocellular adenoma in men. *J. Clin. Ult.* (1989) **17**: 269–274.

Quinn S F & Gosink B B. Characteristic sonographic signs of hepatic fatty infiltration. *Am. J. Roent.* (1985) **45**: 753–755.

Quinn S F *et al.* Torsion of the gall bladder, findings on CT and sonography and role of percutaneous cholecystostomy. *Am. J. Roent.* (1987) **148**: 881–882.

Raby N *et al.* Assessment of portal vein patency: comparison of arterial portography and ultrasound scanning. *Clin. Rad.* (1988) **39**: 381–385.

Radin D R *et al.* Agenesis of the right lobe of liver. *Radiology* (1987) **164**: 639–642.

Raghavencha B N. Ultrasonographic features of primary carcinoma of the gall bladder: report of five cases. *Gastrointest. Radiol.* (1980) **5**: 239–244.

Raghavencha B N *et al.* Acute cholecystitis: sonographic – pathologic analysis. *Am. J. Roent.* (1981) **137**: 327–332.

Ralls P W *et al.* Gall bladder wall thickening: patients without intrinsic gall bladder disease. *Am. J. Roent.* (1981) **137**: 65–68.

Ralls P W *et al.* Real-time sonography in suspected acute cholecystitis. *Radiology* (1985) **155**: 767–771.

Ralls P W *et al.* Greyscale ultrasonography of a

traumatic biliary cyst. *J. Trauma* (1981) **21** (2): 176–177.

Raymond H W & Zwiebel W J. *Seminars Ultrason.* (1982) **1** (2).

Richards D S *et al*. Prenatal diagnosis of fetal liver calcifications. *J. Ult. Med.* (1988) **7**: 691–694.

Roberts J L *et al*. Lipomatous tumours of the liver: evaluation with CT and ultrasound. *Radiology* (1986) **158**: 613–617.

Roemer C E *et al*. Hepatic cysts. Diagnosis and therapy by sonographic needle aspiration. *Am. J. Roent.* (1981) **136**: 1065–1070.

Romano A J *et al*. Gall bladder and bile duct anomalies in Aids: sonographic findings in 8 patients. *Am. J. Roent.* (1988) **150**: 123–127.

Rosenbaum D M & Mindell H J. Ultrasonographic findings in mesenchymal hamartoma of the liver. *Radiology* (1981) **138**: 425–527.

Rutledge J N *et al*. Biliary cystadenoma mistaken for an echinococcal cyst. *South. Med. J.* (1983) **76** (12): 1575–1577.

Saddekni S *et al*. The sonographically patent umbilical vein in portal hypertension. *Radiology* (1982) **145**: 441–443.

Saini S *et al*. Percutaneous aspiration of hepatic cysts does not provide definite therapy. *Am. J. Roent.* (1983) **141**: 559–560.

Sample W *et al*. Greyscale ultrasonography of the jaundiced patient. Presented at the 63rd RSNA meeting 1977.

Sample W F. Techniques for improved delineation of normal anatomy of the upper abdomen and high retroperitoneum with greyscale sound. *Radiology* (1977) **124**: 197–202.

Sanders R C. *Atlas of Ultrasonographic Artefacts and Variants.* Yearbook Medical Publishers (1986) p. 69.

Sanders R C. The significance of sonographic gall bladder wall thickening. *J. Clin. Ult.* (1980) **8**: 143–146.

Sankaran S *et al.* The natural history of pancreatic pseudocysts. *Brit. J. Surg.* (1975) **62**: 37–44.

Sauerbrei E E & Lopaz M. Pseudotumour of the quadrate lobe in hepatic sonography: a sign of generalised fatty infiltration. *Am. J. Roent.* (1986) **147**: 923–927.

Savage P E *et al.* Proceedings of the British Medical Ultrasound Society 17th meeting. *Brit. J. Rad.* (1986) **59**: 703–743.

Sax S L *et al.* Sonographic findings in traumatic haemobilia. *J. Clin. Ult.* (1988) **16**: 29–34.

Schabel S I *et al.* The 'bulls eye' falciform ligament. A sonographic finding of portal hypertension. *Radiology* (1980) **136**: 157–159.

Scheible F & Davis G. Oriental cholangiohepatitis. Preoperative radiographic and sonographic diagnosis. *Gastrointest. Radiol.* (1981) **6**: 269.

Schlaer W J *et al.* Sonography of the thickened gall bladder wall. A non-specific finding. *Am. J. Roent.* (1981) **136**: 337–339.

Schölmerick J & Yolk B A. Differential diagnosis of anechoic/hypoechoic lesions in the abdomen detected by ultrasound. *J. Clin. Ult.* (1986) **14**: 339–353.

Schulman A *et al.* Sonography of biliary worms (ascariasis). *J. Clin. Ult.* (1982) 77–78.

Showker T H *et al.* Distal CBD obstruction, an experimental study on monkeys. *J. Clin. Ult.* (1981) **9**: 77–82.

Simeone J F & Simonds B D. Normal anatomy of the

pancreas by CT and diagnostic ultrasound. In *Clinics in Diagnostic Ultrasound* Vol. 1, pp. 73–84. Churchill Livingstone (1979).

Simeone J F *et al*. Sonography of the bile ducts after a fatty meal: an aid in detection of obstruction. *Radiology* (1982) **143**: 211–215.

Smith R. Carcinoma of the gall bladder and common hepatic duct. In *Surgery of the Gall Bladder and Bile Ducts*, 2nd edn, pp. 393–436. Butterworths (1981).

Solbiali L *et al*. Focal lesions in the spleen: sonographic patterns and guided biopsy. *Am. J. Roent.* (1983) **140**: 59–65.

Spiegel R J & Magrath I T. Tumour lysis pancreatitis. *Med. Paed. Oncol.* (1979) **7**: 169–172.

Spiegel R M *et al*. Ultrasonography of primary cysts of the liver. *Am. J. Roent.* (1978) **131**: 235–238.

Stanley J *et al*. Evaluation of biliary cystadenoma and cystadenocarcinoma. *Gastrointest. Radiol.* (1983) **8**: 245–248.

Stuber *et al*. Sonographic diagnoses of pancreatic lesions. *Am. J. Roent.* (1972) **116**: 406–412.

Swischuk L E & Hayden C K Jr. Pararenal space hyperechogenicity in childhood pancreatitis. *Am. J. Roent.* (1985) **145**: 1085–1086.

Swobodnik W. Ultrasound characteristics of the pancreas in children with cystic fibrosis. *J. Clin. Ult.* (1985) **13**: 469–474.

Takayasu K *et al*. Hepatic lobar atrophy following obstruction of the ipsilateral portal vein from hilar cholangiocarcinoma. *Radiology* (1986) **160**: 389–393.

Tsujmoto F *et al*. Differentiation of benign from malignant ascites by sonographic evaluation of the gall bladder wall. *Radiology* (1985) **157**: 503–504.

Van Sonnenberg E *et al*. Biliary pressure: manometric

and perfusion studies at percutaneous transhepatic cholangiography. *Radiology* (1983) **148**: 41–50.

Wales L R. Desquamated gall bladder mucosa: unusual sign of cholecystitis. *Am. J. Roent.* (1982) **139**: 810–811.

Weaver R M *et al.* Greyscale ultrasonographic evaluation of hepatic cystic disease. *Am. J. Roent.* (1978) **130** (5): 849–852.

Webb *et al.* Greyscale ultrasonography of the portal vein. *Lancet* (1977) **2**: 675–677.

Weiner S N *et al.* Sonography and computed tomography in the diagnosis of carcinoma of the gall bladder. *Am. J. Roent.* (1984) **142**: 735–739.

Weinreb V̄ *et al.* Portal vein measurements by real-time sonography. *Am. J. Roent.* (1982) **139**: 497–499.

Weinstein D P *et al.* Ultrasonic characteristics of pancreatic tumours. *Gastrointest. Radiol.* (1979) **4**: 245–251.

Weinstein D P *et al.* Ultrasonography of biliary tract dilatation without jaundice. *Am. J. Roent.* (1979) **132**: 729–734.

Wellwood J M *et al.* Large intrahepatic cysts and pseudocysts. *Am. J. Surg.* (1978) **135**: 57–64.

White M *et al.* Imaging cholecystocolic fistulas. *J. Ult. Med.* (1983) **2**: 181–185.

Wilson S R *et al.* Leiomyosarcoma of the portal vein. *Am. J. Roent.* (1987) **149**: 183–184.

Wootes W B *et al.* Ultrasonography of necrotic hepatic metastases. *Radiology* (1978) **128**: 447–450.

Yel H C. Ultrasonography and computed tomography of carcinoma of the gall bladder. *Radiology* (1979) **133**: 167–173.

Youngwirth L D *et al.* The suprahepatic gall bladder, an unusual anatomical variant. *Radiology* (1983) **148**: 57–58.

Zorzi C *et al.* Diagnostic value of ultrasonography in neonatal liver rupture. *Paed. Radiol.* (1986) **16**: 425–426.

Chapter 3

Gastrointestinal Tract

3.1 THE OESOPHAGUS

The distal 3 cm of the oesophagus lies within the abdomen having passed through the diaphragm at the level of the 10th thoracic vertebral body. It can usually be identified lying behind the left lobe of liver on the left side of the caudate lobe anterior to the aorta. It is seen as a tube or ring with hypoechoic walls representing the oesophageal wall muscle with a central echogenic band representing the mucosa. The lumen is not usually visualized unless the patient is drinking or there is gastro-oesophageal reflux.

3.1.1 Oesophageal varices

These are seen as multiple anechoic tubes around the distal oesophagus and occur in cases of portal hypertension.

3.1.2 Gastro-oesophageal reflux

Gastro-oesophageal reflux may be diagnosed sonographically but reflux is an intermittent phenomenon and thus examination looking for evidence of reflux must be prolonged. It is also necessary to position the patient so that there is fluid lying over the gastro-oesophageal junction. The examination may start with the patient lying in the supine position but it may be necessary to raise the left side or even place the patient in the head down position to allow reflux to occur. Fluid refluxing into the oesophagus is seen as an anechoic column within the oesophageal lumen. With slight reflux the column is small, transient and easily missed. With more severe reflux the column of fluid is long and may persist for some time. The fluid often contains small echogenic air bubbles caused by turbulent flow. It should be remembered that the tone in the lower oesophageal sphincter is not fully developed until seven weeks of age and reflux before this time is physiological. With care the accuracy of sonography in the diagnosis of gastro-oesophageal reflux is similar to the accuracy of barium meal examination though these two examinations are less accurate than pH probe studies.

Hiatus hernias may occasionally be diagnosed sonographically. They are usually only seen when outlined by fluid and their thoracic extent is not reliably assessed.

3.1.3　Oesophageal tumours

The oesophagus is a frequent site of malignancy particularly in the elderly and this may give rise to a visible mass within or around the oesophageal wall. Tumour spread usually occurs longitudinally along the oesophageal wall and there may be extensive tumour spread without a sonographically detectable mass lesion. In the neonate and young child neurenteric and duplication cysts and other congenital abnormalities may give rise to cystic, complex or solid masses around the oesophagus or bowel.

3.2 THE STOMACH

Conventional scanning of the stomach wall shows two layers. The inner echogenic layer represents the mucosa and submucosa whilst the outer hypoechoic layer represents the gastric muscle. Intra-operative scanning of the stomach wall with a high frequency probe shows five layers, the inner, outer and central layers being echogenic while the remaining two layers are relatively hypoechoic. Intra-operative scanning may prove useful to determine the extent of tumour spread during gastric resection.

When the patient is supine fluid often collects in the gastric fundus which is posterior in position. This is seen as an anechoic collection medial to the spleen and upper pole of the left kidney. Food debris such as milk curds may appear solid and echogenic and may be mistaken for a mass. The pylorus lies anteriorly as it crosses the spine and has a ring or 'bulls eye' appearance in sagittal section. At this point it is anterior to the pancreas and superior mesenteric vein.

3.2.1 The stomach wall

Gastric wall thickness is usually less than 4 mm. Wall thickness of 5 mm or more is highly suspicious of disease though transient wall thickening is seen when the stomach is collapsed or during peristalsis.

A Causes of gastric wall thickening

Tumours. Benign and malignant (primary and secondary)
Lymphoid hyperplasia
Gastric ulceration
Hypertrophic pyloric stenosis

Varioliform gastritis
Henoch–Schonlein purpura
Crohn's disease
Ectopic pancreas
Chronic granulomatous disease of childhood
Haematoma
Focal foveolar hypertrophy

3.2.2 Gastric tumours

Ultrasonography is an unreliable means of demonstrating bowel masses and is thus not the investigation of choice in cases of suspected bowel malignancy. Despite this we visualize bowel tumours from time to time and ultrasonography can be of value at demonstrating totally unsuspected bowel masses particularly those which tend to present late such as caecal carcinoma.

Primary gastric neoplasms are rare in childhood, the commonest being teratomas. These are seen as anechoic or hypoechoic masses which may show evidence of calcification. They usually occur in the first year of life and are found in boys more often than girls. Hamartomas of the gastric wall produce marked wall thickening and protrude into the gastric lumen in a polypoid fashion. This may be mistaken for food residue. Adenocarcinoma of the stomach is rare in children but is common in the elderly. It causes thickening of the gastric wall with a mixed but generally hypoechoic echopattern. Anechoic areas occur due to focal necrosis. Gastric lymphoma and lymphosarcoma give rise to relatively anechoic masses and similar changes occur with leiomyoma and leiomyosarcoma though these tumours may also give rise to complex or multicystic masses. Haematomas of the gastric wall also give rise to anechoic or hypoechoic masses and these are not an uncommon cause of small masses in the stomach wall particularly after endoscopy. They usually occur in the body of stomach and are rare in the pylorus. Sonographic appearances of intramural gastric masses are thus quite non-specific.

3.2.3 Gastric ulceration

Oedema and cellular infiltration of the gastric wall causes thickening which may be echogenic or hypo-echoic. Slight thickening of the underlying muscle may also occur. Unless it is large the ulcer crater cannot usually be visualized and as gastric malignancy often causes ulceration sonography cannot reliably differentiate benign ulcers from tumours.

3.2.4 Gastric duplication cysts

The stomach is an uncommon site for duplication cysts accounting for only 4 % of cases. They are seen as cystic masses which have an inner echogenic layer of mucosa and an outer hypoechoic layer of muscle in their wall. Uncommonly they communicate with the gastric lumen and in these cases the appearance is more complex.

3.2.5 Infantile hypertrophoic pyloric stenosis (HPS)

HPS is a condition characterized by pyloric muscle hypertrophy resulting in gastric outlet obstruction. It is a relatively common condition affecting 1 in 150 boys and 1 in 775 girls. The exact aetiology is uncertain but there appear to be hereditary factors though interestingly it is more common in the children of affected females than affected males. It has also been suggested that trauma caused by the presence of a nasogastric tube in a neonate may also increase the risk of HPS. The pylorus has been shown to be normal at birth and it is thought that the pyloric muscle hypertrophy may occur in response to trauma caused by the passage of milk curds. Spasm induced by this trauma leads to muscle hypertrophy but also increases the pyloric narrowing. HPS is thus not an 'all or nothing' phenomenon but a condition which evolves over a period of time, usually a few days. The majority of cases present in the 2–8 week age group with a history of increasing vomiting which becomes projectile. Gastric peristalsis may be visible and a pyloric muscle mass is usually palpable after a test feed. Five per cent of cases are associated with jaundice which clears after surgery.

In 83 % of cases the findings are sufficiently characteristic to proceed to surgery without any form of imaging. In the remaining 17 % ultrasonography is the investigation of choice to confirm or exclude the diagnosis. It has replaced barium meal examination which has an error rate of up to 10 % in the diagnosis of HPS, this error rate is due to the lack of specificity of barium meal findings which cannot differentiate pylorospasm from true HPS and may also miss early cases. Ultrasonography is also safer and less time consuming than barium meal examination.

On ultrasonography the normal pylorus is seen as a ring of hypoechoic muscle with an inner ring of echogenic mucosa. In HPS there is marked thickening of the pyloric muscle relative to the rest of the stomach and this compresses the mucosa into a single echogenic band. The lumen is only seen in 10 % of cases of HPS and then it is only seen on prolonged scanning when it is visible for a short period of time during the passage of a short 'jet' of fluid. Even when visible the lumen never dilates to its normal calibre. The gallbladder is a good landmark for pyloric location. If the pylorus is still not identified the whole of the upper abdomen should be examined as the pylorus may be displaced to the right lateral abdominal wall or it may be directed posteriorly instead of transversely. If the stomach has not been drained by a nasogastric tube then it will usually be full even 4 h after the last feed or after vomiting. An empty stomach in the absence of vomiting or nasogastric drainage makes HPS unlikely.

Once located the pylorus is evaluated and the muscle compared with that of the body of stomach. In HPS the pylorus assumes a 'doughnut' appearance due to the marked muscle thickening. In some cases the normally hypoechoic muscle may appear anechoic. The mucosa is compressed into a single echogenic band. Pyloric measurements may be a useful aid to diagnosis but when a classic HPS configuration is seen by the experienced sonographer the diagnosis has been made. Lack of visualization of a pyloric muscle mass does not exclude the diagnosis but rather a search should be made for the pylorus and its normality confirmed by demonstration of the normal muscle thickness and full dilatation during the passage of fluid. If these rules are followed there should be no false positive results though false negatives may occur in early cases where pyloric muscle hypertrophy is not fully developed. In cases of doubt the examination is simply repeated on the following day. False positive results may occur if the sonographer relies solely upon measurement of the pyloric dimensions for diagnosis as the pyloric dimensions may be above the normal range when it is transiently dilated during gastric emptying. (In these cases the pyloric configuration is not that of HPS and there is no evidence of a muscle mass.) The great variation in children's sizes even in the neonatal period may cause difficulties when tables of normal values are used in diagnosis.

A Pyloric muscle thickness, (measured from base of echogenic mucosa to outer edge of muscle)

Normal 2.3 ± 0.7 mm
HPS 4.5 ± 0.9 mm

Total pyloric diameter

Normal 7.45 ± 2.2 mm
HPS 13.4 ± 1.6 mm

Pyloric length

Normal 10 − 13.5 mm
HPS 14 − 26 mm

Generally if the muscle thickness is greater than 4 mm or total pyloric diameter is greater than 15 mm then a confident diagnosis of HPS can be made provided a pyloric mass is clearly present. Pyloric haematomas are very rare and are seen as anechoic collections around or adjacent to the muscle. Chronic granulomatous disease of childhood does not usually cause gastric outlet obstruction at such an early age and focal foveolar hypertrophy causes irregular wall thickening with an irregular inner surface without mucosal compression into a single band. If doubt remains after evaluation of the pylorus then the baby should be given fluid either orally or by nasogastric tube and the pylorus evaluated during the passage of this fluid.

3.3 CAUSES OF PYLORIC MASSES IN YOUNG CHILDREN

HPS
Chronic granulomatous disease
Focal foveolar hypertrophy
Focal pyloric haematoma
Gastric duplication cyst
Tumours (very rare in infants) e.g. leiomyoma
    leiomyosarcoma, leiomyoblastoma, lipoma,
    liposarcoma, neurofibroma
Aberrant pancreatic tissue
Hamartoma

3.3.1 Pylorospasm (antral dyskinesia)

Pylorospasm is relatively common in infancy and may cause symptoms similar to HPS but without a palpable pyloric mass. It may be related to vagal overstimulation and hyperacidity. Increased pyloric tone also occurs in association with neurological disorders and these cases are easily mistaken for HPS on barium meal examination. Sonographically the pylorus shows normal muscle thickness but it appears narrowed with ineffective transmission of peristalsis and delayed gastric emptying.

3.3.2 Pseudohypertrophic pyloric stenosis

The pyloric muscle may appear thickened during muscle contraction particularly in the presence of pylorospasm. This is a transient phenomenon which may be exaggerated if the sections through the pylorus are oblique. Imaging the pylorus in several dimensions over a period of time will reveal the transient nature of this finding.

3.3.3 Focal foveolar hyperplasia

Focal foveolar hyperplasia is the commonest cause of gastric polyps in the adult but is rare in infants. These polyps are thought to occur due to hyper-regeneration of mucosa after injury and may be associated with partial gastrectomy, bile reflux and Menetrier's disease. These polyps are usually asymptomatic but have been recorded as a cause of gastric outlet obstruction in neonates. This is seen as a lobulated pyloric mass of similar echogenicity to adjacent mucosa but with normal pyloric muscle.

3.3.4 Chronic granulomatous disease

This is a disorder of phagocytes which are able to engulf bacteria but are unable to kill them. This leads to increased susceptibility to bacterial infection, particularly with staphylococci. It is an inherited condition transmitted as an x-linked or less often as an autosomal recessive trait. Chronic infection leads to granulomatous tissue formation particularly in the lungs, liver and gastric antrum. These granulomata may eventually calcify and become visible on plain radiographs. Involvement of the pyloric antrum causes wall thickening with luminal narrowing. Affected children are usually older than those with HPS and have a slower onset of symptoms. Antibiotic treatment is often successful at relieving gastric outlet obstruction without the need for surgery.

3.3.5 Antropyloric membranes

The presence of membranes across the bowel is a form of focal atresia which is thought to be due to interuterine stress such as anoxia or focal ischaemia. As the bowel heals, scarring causes focal narrowing. Bowel obstruction is usually incomplete due to the presence of a small opening in the membrane. The membrane may be seen as a constant band surrounded by fluid. If a membrane lies in the distal pylorus it is easily mistaken for the division between the pylorus and duodenum.

3.3.6 Pyloric haematomas

Small intra-mural haematomas are common in the oesophagus and stomach particularly after endoscopy. These rarely cause symptoms and are usually not visualized sonographically. Larger haematomas may be recognized as anechoic intramural masses. Large symptomatic haematomas are rare and are often associated with haemorrhagic disease or other underlying pathology. A pyloric haematoma has been recorded causing gastric outlet obstruction in a baby. It was seen as an anechoic ring around normal pyloric muscle and was thus differentiated from HPS.

3.4 THE DUODENUM

The first and second parts of the duodenum are frequently filled with air giving rise to areas of marked echogenicity with distal shadowing and reverberation echoes. Visualization of the duodenal lumen is facilitated by drinking fluids then lying in the right side down position. When distended by fluid the second part of the duodenum defines the lateral aspect of the head of pancreas. The first and upper second parts of the duodenum frequently bulge into the medial side of the distended gallbladder.

3.5 NEONATAL DUODENAL DISTENSION

Duodenal atresia. Double bubble appearance of distended stomach and duodenal cap

Duodenal stenosis

Transient duodenal obstruction of the newborn. (May be a form of superior mesenteric artery syndrome with compression of the fourth part of the duodenum)

Preduodenal portal vein

Oesophageal atresia. (Without tracheo-oesophageal fistula may be associated with a fluid filled duodenal loop)

Midgut volvulus

Annular pancreas

Duodenal/proximal jejunal haematoma

Secondary to proximal small bowel obstruction

Duodenal bands. Ladd's bands may compress and obstruct the third and fourth parts of the duodenum. They are usually associated with malrotation which predisposes to

> midgut volvulus. An upper GI barium series
> is the most reliable means of confirming
> the diagnosis which requires urgent surgery
> Paraduodenal hernia. Rare condition in which
> the duodenum is herniated internally
> through the mesenteric origin

3.5.1 Malrotation

Malrotation of the bowel occurs when the distal limb of the developing midgut fails to rotate on returning to the abdomen. The normal midgut undergoes a total rotation of 270° to achieve its final configuration. Malrotation is a spectrum of congenital abnormalities ranging from reverse rotation and non-rotation of bowel to lesser degrees of rotation in which the bowel has failed to rotate the full 270°. Mild cases are not uncommon and simply result in a high placed caecum. More severe cases are uncommon but potentially fatal as malrotation is often associated with a short small bowel mesentery origin which predisposes to volvulus. This causes acute bowel ischaemia which, without urgent surgery causes bowel infarction. Sonographically malrotation with volvulus may be identified by alteration in the normal relationship of the superior mesenteric artery and vein. The vein normally lies on the right of the artery but this relationship may be reversed. In lesser degrees of malrotation alterations in vascular anatomy may not be so clear and thus in any suspected case a barium examination should be performed as delayed diagnosis may be fatal. In our experience though ultrasonography is valuable at showing altered vascular anatomy the mesenteric vessels are obscured by bowel gas in the majority of acute cases with volvulus. We have recently shown that normal mesenteric vascular anatomy does not exclude malrotation as a cause of bilous vomiting in children.

3.5.2 Duodenal haematomas

The duodenum is retroperitoneal throughout most of its course and is fixed and thus relatively prone to injury. Haematomas are not uncommon particularly after blunt abdominal injury and are seen as anechoic intramural collections which are usually eccentric. They may remain anechoic or become echogenic. Large haematomas may cause bowel obstruction but usually resolve over a few weeks. If a duodenal haematoma is encountered without a suitable history of trauma or underlying abnormality the possibility of non-accidental injury should be considered.

3.5.3 Duodenal duplication cysts

The duodenum is an uncommon site for duplication cysts, they occur more frequently in the oesophagus and distal small bowel. Sonographically they are seen as cystic structures usually within the C of the duodenal loop.

3.6 DUODENAL WALL THICKENING

Haematoma
Pancreatitis
Post bulbar duodenal ulcer
Adjacent varices – seen as a 'cluster of grape-
like anechoic structures' or a 'bag of
worms'
Osler–Rendu–Weber syndrome
Retroperitoneal haemangioma
Retroperitoneal abscess. In children
periduodenal abscess or haematoma should
raise the possibility of non-accidental injury.
In adults abscesses are usually due to
duodenal ulceration
Duodenal duplication
Inflammatory bowel disease

3.7 JEJUNUM AND ILEUM

Small bowel visualization is improved when it is fluid
filled. This may occur in normal individuals particularly
after meals or the injection of large volumes of fluids.
Sonography shows fluid-filled tubes lined by echogenic
mucosa which is thrown into folds or valvulae. These
may give the inner wall a ribbed appearance. The
normal small bowel wall thickness is 3–5 mm. Normal
loops are compliant and are easily deformed during
examination. They may alter configuration during
waves of peristalsis. Ileus leads to loss of peristalsis with
distention of bowel loops by fluid and air. Progressive
distention makes the bowel more tubular with loss of
the sharp angles through which loops may normally
turn.

3.7.1 Features of small bowel obstruction

Bowel loop distension

Loops have a rounded contour and show little deformity due to adjacent bowel loops

Loss of definition and loss of prominence of valvulae conniventes

Variable peristalsis. Distended bowel becomes paralysed and thus bowel close to the site of obstruction may be aperistaltic

Variation in peristalsis may make it difficult to differentiate ileus from obstruction. Peristalsis is reduced or absent in ileus but peristalsis is frequently reduced or absent in bowel immediately proximal to an obstruction

A *Sonographic features of fluid-filled bowel*

DUODENUM – Fluid filled bowel has a 'keyboard' or 'step ladder' configuration. Fluid column may contain debris and may be continuous with the stomach.

JEJUNUM – Bowel is tubular with a 'keyboard' margin due to valvulae conniventes.

ILEUM – Fluid filled bowel is smoother and more featureless than proximal small bowel.

COLON – Generally the colon is peripherally situated in the abdomen whilst the small bowel is more centrally placed. Ascending and transverse colon show haustral sacculations. The descending colon has a more tubular appearance and the rectum lies deep in the pelvis behind the bladder.

3.8 CAUSES OF SMALL BOWEL WALL THICKENING

Hypoalbuminaemia/hypoproteinaemia
Sprue
Protein loosing enteropathy
Cancer chemotherapy
Ischaemia and intramural haemorrhage
Venous congestion including malrotation and
    chronic volvulus
Intestinal lymphangiectasia
Henoch Schonlein purpura (may accentuate
    the mucosal pattern)
Pelvic inflammatory disease ⎫
Appendix abscess   ⎬ Changes usually focal
Trauma   ⎭
Crohn's disease. Concentric thickening of the
    bowel wall with narrowing of the lumen.
    The bowel wall may be of reduced
    echogenicity
Eosinophilic enteritis
Amyloidosis
Mastocytosis
Whipple's disease
Giardiasis/strongyloidiasis
Behcets syndrome. Appearances similar to
    Crohn's
Radiation. Bowel wall thickening with
    thickening of the valvulae conniventes
    (stacked coin appearance)
Lymphoma. Eccentric bowel wall thickening by
    lymphomatous infiltrate. This is usually
    anechoic but haemorrhage and clot may
    give rise to echogenic areas. There may be

aneurysmal dilatation of the bowel lumen and enlargement of adjacent lymph nodes. Anechoic deposits may mimic duplication cysts. The combination of eccentric bowel wall thickening with aneurysmal dilatation and mesenteric lymphadenopathy produces the so called 'sandwich' sign which distinguishes lymphoma from Crohn's disease.

Dermatomyositis and collagen vascular disease. These cause bowel wall thickening with reduced peristalsis

Abscess

Necrotizing enterocolitis

Amoebiasis

Pseudomembranous colitis

Adenocarcinoma

Tumours including metastases

Pneumatosis intestinalis (intramural high amplitude echoes with shadowing)

Kaposi's sarcoma

3.8.1 Abnormal bowel patterns

The jejunum is wider than the ileum and has thicker walls with more circular mucosal folds than the ileum. In the distal ileum the mucosal folds become longitudinal. These appearances are normal findings and should not be mistaken for pathology. The non-distended small bowel loop gives a target appearance with hypoechoic muscular walls in transverse section. The muscle is lined by an echogenic layer representing the mucosa and submucosa. Gas within the bowel lumen frequently prevents visualization of the distal bowel wall and underlying structures.

a) Thickening of the sonolucent halo (bowel wall). Exact measurement of bowel wall thickness is unreliable owing to the great variation in apparent wall thickness with bowel distension and peristalsis. Slight thickening of the bowel wall is usually missed but marked thickening is usually obvious

b) Asymmetric location of the echogenic mucosal band indicating irregular bowel wall thickening. Asymmetric bowel wall thickening or the 'atypical target' appearance is a non-specific appearance but it is indicative of bowel pathology

c) Lack of change in configuration or peristalsis on prolonged imaging

d) Irregular bowel contour

3.9 ATYPICAL TARGET CONFIGURATION OF BOWEL

Bowel usually has a 'ring like' or target appearance. 'Atypical target' apearance due to asymmetric bowel wall thickening occurs in:

Adenocarcinoma
Lymphosarcoma
Leiomyosarcoma
Intussusception
Crohn's disease
Amyloidosis
Whipples disease
Intramural haematoma
Serosal implants
Appendicitis
Pneumatosis coli/intestinalis

3.9.1 Jejunal and ileal duplication cysts

Duplication cysts occur more frequently in the jejunum and ileum than any other segment of bowel. They usually do not communicate with the bowel lumen and are seen as anechoic structures which may be indistinguishable from mesenteric and peritoneal cysts. The cyst wall is usually hypoechoic with an echogenic lining. They can contain ectopic gastric and pancreatic tissue which may bleed and perforate.

3.9.2 Meckel's diverticulum

Meckel's diverticulum is a remnant of the proximal end of the vitello-intestinal duct of the embryo. It is found in 2–3 % of the population but rarely causes symptoms. It lies on the anti-mesenteric border of the distal ileum 30–50 cm from the caecum and is 3–6 cm long. Symptoms may arise when the diverticulum contains ectopic gastric or pancreatic tissue which may secrete acid or enzymes causing ulceration and haemorrhage. These diverticula are rarely visible sonographically but have been noted when distended with fluid.

3.9.3 Meconium ileus

Sonography may demonstrate ecogenic meconium within the dilated distal bowel lumen thus confirming the diagnosis.

3.9.4 Inflammatory bowel disease

Infective enteritis may give rise to transient small bowel changes but Crohn's disease is the commonest chronic inflammatory disease of small bowel. Eighty per cent of cases involve distal ileum whilst disease is limited to the colon in 10 % of cases at presentation. The incidence of Crohn's disease has risen in recent years and 20 % of cases are diagnosed in childhood. Ultrasonography may demonstrate small bowel changes such as focal or generalized bowel wall thickening, bowel masses, rigid loops, abscesses etc. In longstanding cases fibrosis results in stiff, thick, echogenic, illdefined bowel walls. Though ultrasonography is unreliable in the detection of bowel pathology a review of the mid and lower abdomen may be rewarding in patients with symptoms suggesting small bowel disease.

3.9.5 Intestinal lymphangiectasia

Intestinal lymphangiectasia is a rare lymphatic disorder in which obstruction of lymph drainage causes lymphatic stasis within the bowel wall and mucosal congestion. The bowel wall and mucosa are thickened and may weep proteinaceous fluid causing malabsorption or protein loosing enteropathy. Fluid filled lacteals may give rise to anechoic spaces but these are rarely seen and the sonographic pattern is usually a non-specific picture of diffuse small bowel wall thickening. Identical appearances have been recorded in children with malrotation and chronic volvulus, venous congestion, Crohn's and other inflammatory bowel diseases. It is said that the bowel is less rigid in lymphatic congestion than portal venous congestion allowing transmission of peristaltic waves but assessment is subjective.

3.9.6 Small bowel tumours

Small bowel tumours are uncommon in adults and relatively rare in children. Benign tumours may be

polypoid and may form part of a polyposis syndrome
e.g. Peutz–Jegher's syndrome. Malignant tumours may
be primary or secondary to almost any distant tumour.
The commonest primary tumour in childhood is
lymphosarcoma or Burkitt's lymphoma. In adults
metastases are more common particularly in the elderly
e.g. from carcinoma of the bronchus. Small bowel
tumours are frequently not visualized sonographically.
When seen they may have a mass or target appearance.
The mass may lie within the bowel lumen or replace
the bowel wall. There is usually a thick sonolucent
rim though the overall pattern may be heterogenous.
Luminal small bowel tumours may cause intussusception giving rise to a mass with a layered appearance.
Small bowel obstruction may occur causing dilatation
of the proximal small bowel with fluid and gas-filled
bowel loops.

3.10 THE LARGE BOWEL

The large bowel usually contains air and is thus not clearly visualized sonographically in the majority of cases. Despite this sonography can give valuable information in a variety of circumstances.

3.10.1 Appendicitis

Appendicitis is the second most frequent inflammatory process within the abdomen, gastroenteritis being the most common. It is relatively rare in infancy but is common in children and young adults. Appendicitis occurs when obstruction of the appendix lumen causes a build up of secretions. This stretches the wall causing ischaemia. In the presence of bacterial infection the inflamed appendix may perforate as early as 6 h after the onset of symptoms and the risk of perforation with resultant peritonitis increases with time.

If the right iliac fossa is not obscured by bowel gas and the patient can tolerate the examination ultrasonography may confirm the diagnosis of appendicitis in patients whose symptoms are not sufficiently prominent to warrant urgent surgery. With care 89 % of inflamed appendices can be visualized and perforation can be predicted in 80 % of cases. The inflamed appendix is seen as a non-compressible aperistaltic tubular structure. In transverse section it has the typical target appearance of bowel. The central dilated lumen varies from 6 to 20 mm, (mean 8 mm). This is surrounded by a thin echogenic mucosal layer and an outer hypoechoic layer representing oedematous muscle. Faecoliths may be seen within the lumen as echogenic foci with shadowing. Further signs include fluid around the appendix, an inflammatory bowel mass and abscess formation. Thirty per cent of cases have demonstrable lymphadenopathy in the adjacent mesentery.

In the majority of cases appendicitis remains a clinical diagnosis but sonography is valuable in the assessment of complications such as abscess formation. The majority of abscesses secondary to appendicitis occur in the pelvis or right iliac fossa though pus may spread to the psoas muscle, subhepatic space or either subphrenic space. Intra-abdominal inflammation may also give rise to portal vein thrombosis and liver abscess both of which may be demonstrated sonographically.

3.10.2 Appendix abscess

Abscesses are not uncommon in appendicitis particularly if surgery was delayed or the appendix ruptured. Abscesses usually lie in the pelvis or right iliac fossa and are seen as irregular anechoic collections. Small collections are easily mistaken for bowel loops and in cases of doubt the examination should be repeated after an interval to allow bowel loops to change configuration. Large collections can be clearly identified as extra-luminal and may contain debris.

3.10.3 Mucocoele of the appendix

Progressive cystic dilatation of the appendix due to obstruction of the lumen may occur without bacterial infection. In these cases accumulation of mucus may give rise to a cystic right iliac fossa mass. The majority of cases are due to the presence of a faecolith or inflammatory stricture but 10 % of cases are secondary to malignancy (usually mucinous cystadenocarcinoma of appendix). Rupture of the mucocoele may lead to pseudomyxoma peritoneii.

A Appearances

A cystic mass extrinsic to solid abdominal organs

Highly echogenic mass due to fine calcification

Mucosal hypertrophy, adherent debris and tumour nodules may give rise to nodules on the inner wall of the mucocoele

Multiseptate mucocoeles have been described on CT and will presumably be demonstrable sonographically

Mobile dependent echoes may occur due to the presence of debris or protein macroaggregates

A mucocoele may appear heterogenous without distal enhancement particularly if the iliac wing is directly posterior

Pseudomyxoma peritoneii may also be demonstrated sonographically, appearances are similar to ascites but the bowel loops may be depressed by the mucus rather than floating in it and scalloping of the hepatic outline has also been recorded. Septae may also be seen within the mucinous collection.

3.10.4 Intussusception

Intussusception is the invagination or herniation of a segment of bowel into an adjacent segment of bowel in a manner analogous to the shortening of a telescope. The majority of cases occur in children and of these cases 95 % involve the passage of ileum into the caecum and colon (ileo-colic). In children 75 % of cases occur in boys, frequency is highest in spring and autumn and lymphoid inflammation is thought to play a part in the origin of the intussusception. The diagnosis is usually suspected clinically as the patient develops bowel obstruction with colic and vomiting. The child may in addition pass 'redcurrant jelly' stool. Five per cent of childhood cases have an underlying abnormality at the apex of the intussusception such as a polyp, Meckel's diverticulum, hamartoma, Crohn's, Henoch Schonlein purpura or tumour. This incidence of underlying pathology is much higher in adult cases.

Sonographically the intussusception is seen as a bowel mass with multiple concentric echogenic rings produced by alternating mucosal and muscular layers. This has been described as a 'doughnut' appearance on transverse section and 'pseudokidney' appearance on longitudinal section. The outer rim is usually relatively sonolucent due to oedema whilst the centre of the mass may show one or more layers of echogenic infolded mucosa. A similar appearance can be seen with bowel tumours but these usually give a different history. Other reported causes of these appearances include necrotizing enterocolitis, volvulus and inflammatory bowel disease. Hydrostatic reduction has been attempted under ultrasound control and it has been said that the greater the echogenicity of the central mucosal band the greater will be the difficulty of reduction. It is felt that a narrow central mucosal band reflects greater mucosal compression. Though ultrasonography is a reliable means of diagnosing intussusception its accuracy is not as great as that of a barium enema. Also, monitoring reduction by ultrasonography is not as accurate as radiography and thus we prefer diagnosis and therapy by traditional methods.

3.10.5 Inflammatory disease of the colon

Excluding infective and toxic states Crohn's disease and ulcerative colitis are the commonest causes of chronic large bowel inflammation. Sonographic features are non-specific and include bowel-wall thickening which may involve both the hypoechoic muscular coat and the echogenic mucosa. Localized perforation may occur leading to abscess formation which may be clinically silent if the patient is receiving steroid therapy.

3.10.6 Ischaemic bowel disease

Bowel ischaemia is mainly a disease of old age caused by atheroma of the mesenteric vessels. Bowel gas frequently prevents visualization of colonic changes which are usually most marked around the splenic flexure. In the initial stages the ischaemic bowel may show increased peristalsis which is then reduced. The bowel wall becomes thickened and nodular and intramural haemorrhage and oedema give rise to areas of reduced echogenicity. Echogenic areas may develop in the bowel wall and these may reflect either areas of infarction, infiltrate or clot. Echogenic areas with shadowing occur due to the presence of intramural gas. Gas in the portal vein also occurs and is associated with a very poor prognosis in adults.

3.10.7 Necrotizing enterocolitis

Necrotizing enterocolitis is an inflammatory disorder which occurs mainly in pre-term infants though it can affect full-term infants usually in the epidemic form of the disease. Aetiology is multifactorial. Hypoxia induces vasospasm and thus intestinal ischaemia. This reduces intestinal mucosal integrity and resistance to bacteria. Initially the ischaemic bowel is paralysed causing gaseous distension. The bowel wall is thickened and gas may penetrate the wall. In severe cases the gas may enter the portal venous system and the bowel may perforate causing peritonitis. Sonographically the bowel may be obscured by the large volume of gas present. When visible there is exaggeration of the normal target or bull's eye appearance due to bowel wall thickening. High amplitude intramural echoes with distal shadowing may occur due to the presence of intramural air. Portal venous gas is seen as high amplitude echoes within the peripheral portal vein radicles in the liver. Ultrasonography may show these changes before any abnormality is evident on the plain abdominal radiograph.

3.10.8 Colonic neoplasms

Ultrasonography may detect colonic neoplasms which are not palpable and may also be used to locate the site or confirm the presence of a palpable abdominal mass. The false positive diagnosis of an abdominal mass by sonography is uncommon but once a mass is demonstrated its appearance is frequently non-specific. Colonic neoplasms give rise to mass lesions with a thickened hypoechoic outer wall which may be heterogenous and a central cluster of echoes due to mucosal compression. Larger tumours may show a more heterogenous appearance and appearances may alter if the tumour extends outside the bowel wall or is predominantly intraluminal.

3.11 COLONIC MASSES WITH A THICKENED BOWEL WALL

Colonic carcinoma
Inflammatory bowel disease
Bowel infarction
Intramural haematoma
Diverticular mass/abscess
Metastases
Lymphoma

FURTHER READING

Avni E *et al.* Sonographic demonstration of malabsorption in the neonate. *J. Ult. Med.* (1986) **5**: 85–87.

Ball T L *et al.* Ultrasound diagnosis of hypertrophic pyloric stenosis: real-time application and the demonstration of a new radiological sign. *Radiology* (1983) **147**: 499–502.

Bisset R *et al.* Radiographic and sonographic appearances of an intramural haematoma of the pylorus. *Clin. Rad.* (1988) **39**: 316–318.

Bisset R A L & Gupta S C. Hypertrophic pyloric stenosis: ultrasonic appearances in a small baby. *Paed. Rad.* (1988) **18**: 405.

Blumhagen J D *et al.* Sonographic diagnosis of hypertrophic pyloric stenosis. *Am. J. Roent.* (1988) **150**: 1367–1370.

Bowerman R A *et al.* Real-time ultrasound diagnosis of intussusception in children. *Radiology* (1982) **143**: 527–529.

Dachmann A H *et al.* Review: mucocoele of the appendix and pseudomyxoma peritonei. *Am. J. Roent.* (1985) **144**: 923–929.

Derchi C E *et al.* Ultrasonographic appearances of gastric cancer. *Brit. J. Rad.* (1983) **56**: 365–370.

Dinkle E *et al.* Real-time ultrasound of Crohn's disease, characteristic features and clinical implications. *Paed. Rad.* (1986) **16**: 131–134.

Fleischer A C *et al.* Sonographic patterns arising from normal and abnormal bowel. *Rad. Clin. North Am.* (1980) **18**(1): 145–159.

Fleischer A C *et al.* Sonographic assessment of the bowel wall. *Am. J. Roent.* (1981) **136**: 887–891.

Fleischer A C *et al.* Real-time sonography of the bowel, *Clinics in Diagnostic Ultrasound* (1982): 117–135.

Fon V T *et al.* Utility of ultrasound for the diagnosis of mesenteric haematoma. *Am. J. Roent.* (1980) **134**: 381–384.

Fried A W *et al.* Duodenal duplication cysts, sonographic and angiographic features. *Am. J. Roent.* (1977) **128**: 863–865.

Jackson G H *et al.* Sonography of combined oesophageal duodenal atresia. *J. Ult. Med.* (1983) **2**: 473–474.

Jeffrey R B *et al.* Acute appendicitis: high resolution real-time ultrasound findings. *Radiology* (1987) **163**: 11–14.

Kodroff M B *et al.* Ultrasonographic diagnosis of gangrenous bowel in neonatal necrotising enterocolitis. *Paed. Rad.* (1984) **14**: 168–171.

Kurtz A B & Goldberg B B eds, *Clinics in Diagnostic Ultrasound* 23: *Gastrointestinal Ultrasonography*. Churchill Livingstone (1988).

Li Y P *et al.* Ultrasound findings in mucocoele of the appendix. *J. Clin. Ult.* (1981) **9**: 406.

Limberg B. Diagnosis of acute ulcerative colitis and colonic Crohn's disease by colonic sonography. *J. Clin. Ult.* (1989) **17**: 25–31.

Lindley S *et al.* Portal vein ultrasonography in the early diagnosis of necrotising enterocolitis. *J. Paed. Surg.* (1986) **21**: 53–532.

Malin G W *et al.* Echogenic intravascular and hepatic microbubbles associated with necrotising enterocolitis. *J. Paeds.* (1983) **103**: 637–640.

McAlister W M *et al.* Sonography of focal foveolar hyperplasia causing gastric obstruction in an infant. *Paed. Rad.* (1988) **18**(1): 79.

Miller J H & Kemberling C R. Ultrasound of the paediatric gastrointestinal tract. Seminars in Ultrasound, CT & MR (1987) **8**(4): 349–365.

Miller J H *et al.* Ultrasound in the evaluation of small bowel lymphoma in children. *Radiology* (1980) **135**: 409–414.

Miyamoto Y *et al.* Ultrasonographic findings in gastric cancer: *in vitro* and *in vivo* studies. *J. Clin. Ult.* (1989) **17**: 309–318.

Miyamoto Y *et al.* Ultrasonographic findings in duodenum caused by Schönlein–Henoch purpura. *J. Clin. Ult.* (1989) **17**: 299–303.

Morimotok *et al.* Ultrasonographic evaluation of intramural gastric and duodenal haematoma in haemophiliacs. *J. Clin. Ult.* (1988) **16**: 108–113.

Mueller P R *et al.* Appearances of lymphomatous involvement of the mesentery by ultrasonography and body computed tomography. 'The sandwich sign.' *Radiology* (1980) **134**: 467–473.

Naik D R & Moore D J. Ultrasound diagnosis of gastro-oesophageal reflux. *Arch. Dis. Child.* (1984) **59**: 366–367.

Nicolet V *et al.* Sonographic appearance of an abdominal cystic lymphangioma. *J. Ult. Med.* (1984) **3**: 85–86.

Orel *et al.* Duodenal haematoma in child abuse: sonographic detection. *Am. J. Roent.* (1988) **151**: 147–149.

Pandher D & Sauerbrei E E. Neonatal ileocolic intussusception with enterogenous cysts: ultrasound diagnosis. *J. Can. Ass. Rad.* (1983) **34**: 328–330.

Pearson R H. Ultrasonography for diagnosing appendicitis. Better than other methods but not for routine use. *Brit. Med. J.* (1988) **297**: 309–310.

Pozniak M A *et al.* Ultrasound in the evaluation of bowel disorders. Seminars in ultrasound, CT & MR (1987) **8**(4): 366–384.

Pracrus J P *et al.* Ultrasound diagnosis of intussusception. *Lancet* (1985) **2**: 733–735.

Saverymutty S H *et al.* Ultrasound detection of oesophageal varices – comparison with endoscopy. *Clin. Rad.* (1988) **39**: 513–515.

Schuster M M & Smith V M. The pyloric 'cervix' sign in adult hypertrophic pyloric stenosis. *Gastrointest. Endosc.* (1970) **16**: 210–211.

Schwimer S R *et al.* Unusual presentation of a mucocoele of the appendix. *J. Ult. Med.* (1987) **6**: 85–87.

Seshul M B & Coulam C M. Pseudomyxoma peritonei: computed tomography and sonography. *Am. J. Roent.* (1981) **136**: 803–806.

Sherman *et al.* Sonography in the neonate. *Ult. Quart.* (1988) **6**(2): 91–150.

Stringer D A *et al.* Sonography of the normal and abnormal stomach (excluding hypertrophic pyloric stenosis) in children. *J. Ult. Med.* (1986) **5**: 183–188.

Stringer D A *et al.* Behcet's syndrome involving the gastrointestinal tract – a diagnostic dilemma in childhood. *Paed. Rad.* (1986) **16**: 131–134.

Takada T *et al.* Ultrasonic diagnosis of acute appendicitis complicated by paralytic ileus and generalised peritonitis. *J. Clin. Ult.* (1988) **16**: 123–126.

Vernacchia F S *et al.* Sonographic recognition of pneumatosis intestinalis. *Am. J. Roent.* (1985) **145**: 51–52.

Wilson D A & Vanhoutle J J. The reliable sonographic diagnosis of hypertrophic pyloric stenosis. *J. Clin. Ult.* (1984) **12**: 201–204.

Wing-Kay C *et al.* Real-time ultrasound diagnosis of intramural intestinal haematoma. *J. Clin. Ult.* (1989) **17**: 382–384.

Chapter 4

Urinary tract and adrenal glands

4.1 INTRODUCTION

Anomalies of the genitourinary tract are common and are found in 10% of infants. This high incidence of anatomical variants is explained by the complex embryology of the region. The genital and urinary tracts arise from the urogenital ridges on the posterior abdominal wall. Three pairs of renal structures form in early foetal life, the pronephros (forekidney) and mesonephros (midkidney) involute but the metanephros (hindkidney) which begins to form during the fifth week of life persists to form the definitive kidney which produces urine from the eleventh week of life. The large number of anatomical variants occurs due to anomalies of growth and fusion of the metanephric duct which forms the renal collecting system and ureter and the metanephric mesenchyme which forms the nephrons. The kidneys initially form in the pelvis but differential rates of growth in the length of the trunk cause them to migrate into the abdomen. The renal hilum which is initially directed anteriorly rotates medially as the kidney ascends. Whilst in the pelvis the kidney derives its blood supply from the sacral and iliac vessels but as they ascend into the abdomen they derive their blood supply from the aorta. This changing vascular anatomy accounts for the high incidence of variants encountered – 25 % of patients have three or more renal arteries and this should be remembered when performing angiography.

Anomalies of the kidney and ureter are common affecting 4 % of the population:

The majority of people have two kidneys but unilateral renal agenesis occurs at a rate of 1 case per 1000 population. (Renal fossa may contain bowel loops which may be mistaken for a kidney, abscess or calculus. The adrenal gland is relatively large in the neonate and may be mistaken for a small kidney.)

If a kidney cannot be found search for an ectopic kidney and consider an isotope scan.

Unilateral renal hypoplasia is more common than agenesis. The kidney is small but of normal smooth echopattern and configuration. The main differential diagnosis is ischaemic atrophy but identical appearances can occur with growth retardation due to infection thus renal hypoplasia should not be diagnosed until the urinary tract has been fully evaluated.

Unilateral renal agenesis is frequently associated with other anomalies, particularly in women. Fifty-eight per cent have other congenital anomalies and 48 % of these are of the genital tract e.g. bicornuate uterus, unicornuate uterus, uterine and vaginal septations.

Bilateral renal agenesis (Potter's syndrome) occurs at a rate of 0.3 per 1000 population. It is associated with oligohydramnios, pulmonary hypoplasia and is fatal soon after birth.

Rotational anomalies of the kidneys are uncommon. Rotation normally occurs as the kidney ascends from the pelvis and thus the majority of cases are associated with low or ectopic kidneys. Ectopic kidneys usually lie in the pelvis due to failure of ascent. These kidneys may be malformed due to lack of pressure from adjacent organs during growth. Crossed renal ectopia occurs when a kidney crosses the midline during ascent. In these cases the ureter enters the bladder on the side the kidney originated from.

Renal fusion across the midline results in the formation of a horseshoe kidney. This is found in 1 in 400–600 of the population and in over 90 % of cases renal fusion is at the lower poles. Ascent of the horseshoe kidney is arrested by the mesenteric vessels and thus they are lower in the abdomen than normal. The isthmus joining the two kidneys is often hidden by bowel gas and thus the diagnosis of horseshoe kidney is easily missed on sonography though the kidneys may be noted to have more vertical axes than normal.

Duplications of the renal collecting system and ureter are common affecting 1 in 70 of the population. They occur due to varying degrees of division of the ureteric bud (metanephric diverticulum) as it grows into the urogenital ridge. There is a great variation in the degree of division resulting in a spectrum of changes from completely double collecting system with two ureters to a slightly bifid collecting system draining to a single ureter. Supernumerary kidneys are due to the formation of an extra ureteric bud and are extremely rare. In mild cases the kidney appears normal sonographically but more prominent cases are associated with increased renal length and division of the central echo-complex into two parts on longitudinal sections. This appearance may be mimicked by oblique sections through a normal kidney, renal cysts or renal columnar hypertrophy. When the two renal moieties drain by separate ureters the ureter draining the lower collecting system inserts into the bladder at the normal site but has a shortened intramural course and is prone to reflux. The ureter draining the upper half of the kidney inserts into the bladder distal to the normal site and may insert ectopically into vagina, urethra, seminal vesicles etc. These ureters are prone to ureterocoele formation and obstruction. Ectopic ureteric insertion may also occur less commonly without ureteric duplication.

The urinary bladder forms from the cloaca which divides into the urogenital sinus anteriorly and the rectum posteriorly. The urogenital sinus gives rise to the bladder and urethra and is continuous superiorly with the allantois. The allantois is a diverticulum on the caudal wall of the yolk sac, it extends from the bladder into the placenta and though it normally involutes it may give rise to cysts, fistulae and even tumours such as embryonal rhabdomyosarcoma.

The kidneys are retroperitoneal organs lying obliquely on the posterior abdominal wall. Average renal weight is 150 g in the male and 135 g in the female. The kidney is usually 10–11 cm long, 5 cm wide and 3 cm thick though renal size depends upon the patient's size and build. The kidney is bean shaped with a central concavity or hilum on its medial border which receives the renal vein, artery and pelvis from anterior to posterior. It should be remembered that small vessels may pass around the renal pelvis and upper ureter and may not follow this anatomical relationship. The kidneys are very vascular organs and together receive 25 % of the resting cardiac output, approximately 1250 ml of blood per minute. The renal substance is divided into outer cortex and inner medullary pyramids. Projections of cortex, the columns or septae of Bertin, lie between the pyramids. The collecting system, vessels, nerves, fat and connective tissue lie at the centre of the kidney.

A Sonographic appearances

The sonographic appearances of internal renal anatomy are remarkably similar to the appearance of cut sections of a kidney at post mortem (Fig. 13). Cortical thickness is usually uniform but may be lobulated particularly in neonates. The renal cortex is normally hypoechoic relative to hepatic or splenic parenchyma and renal pyramids are hypoechoic relative to the cortex. The corticomedullary junction is demarcated by the arcuate arteries which are seen as small echogenic foci. The collecting system, vessels and connective tissue at the centre of the kidney are seen as the echogenic 'central echo complex' which is the most echogenic part of the kidney. The echogenicity of the central echo complex increases with age and in conditions such as renal

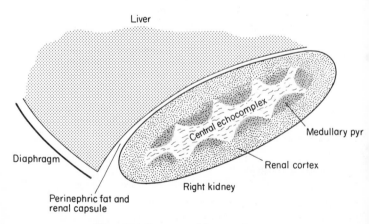

Fig. 13. Sonographic renal anatomy.

fibrolipomatosis. Its echogenicity is reduced in neonates and conditions with reduced total body fat such as starvation.

4.1.1 Normal renal lobulation

FOETAL LOBULATION – Lobulation of the renal contour conforms to renal lobular architecture. This is most prominent in neonates and *in utero* and decreases with age. It may be visible when the kidney is swollen.

DROMEDARY HUMP – Lobulation of the lateral aspect of the left kidney at the site of impression by the lower pole of the spleen occurs due to pressure *in utero* during renal development. It is seen more frequently on sonography than on urography due to the increased number of sections taken.

HYPERTROPHY OF THE RENAL SINUS MARGIN – Prominent renal sinus margin usually seen on transverse sections.

ANTERIOR INDENTATION ON SAGITTAL SECTIONS – This is seen at the level of the renal hilum on sagittal sections and should not be mistaken for pyelonephritic scarring.

OBLIQUE SECTIONS – Sections taken obliquely through the kidney may give the appearance of variation in renal parenchymal thickness. The true cause of this appearance will be evident on further sections.

4.1.2 Renal examination

A Renal location

Locating the kidneys is not always easy particularly in patients with spinal deformity. Do not assume that an atypical structure in the renal bed is a kidney, it could be a bowel loop. If a typically reniform structure is not seen in the renal bed search for ectopic kidneys. When in doubt do a DMSA isotope scan.

B When the kidney is located assess

Position
Mobility
Size
Contour
Parenchymal echopattern
Central echo complex/collecting system
Adjacent structures including the renal artery, vein
   pelvis and perinephric space

4.1.3 Renal size

Renal size may be assessed visually or by direct measurement. The bipolar diameter is the most frequently used parameter measuring from the upper to the lower renal poles. If the sections taken are oblique the bipolar diameter will underestimate the renal length. The greatest measurement obtained for each kidney is the closest estimation of the true renal length. The renal size is related to age, weight and body surface area.

A Renal length

Baby <1 year of age:
Average renal length = 4.98 + (0.155 × age in
                              months) cm
Children >1 year in age:
Average renal length = 6.79 + (0.22 × age in
                              years) cm

Renal length (cm)

Age	5 %	50 %	95 %
		Percentile	
Birth	4	5	6
1 year	5	6.5	8
5 years		8	
10 years	7	9	10.5
Adult	9.5	11	12.5

In infants under one year of age renal size correlates most closely with weight and length thus small babies can be expected to have small kidneys. At birth the two kidneys are approximately the same length but as they grow the left kidney becomes slightly longer and thinner than the right. In older children renal length correlates better with height, weight and surface area than with age.

B Renal volume

Renal volume = width $\times$ length $\times$ thickness $\times$ 0.5233 cm^3

Renal volume

Birth	20 cm^3
1 year	30 cm^3
18 years	155 cm^3

4.1.4 Renal parenchyma

The renal parenchymal echopattern is compared with adjacent organs. Renal cortex is normally less echogenic than liver parenchyma except in the newborn. For the first six months of life the renal cortex may be as echogenic as liver parenchyma. (Fifty per cent of neonatal left kidneys are as echogenic as the spleen.) It has been said that normal neonatal renal cortex is never more echogenic than liver though there are reports of very echogenic cortex in the kidneys of pre-term infants. If there is doubt about the normality of the parenchyma of a neonatal kidney it should be followed up as 90 % of infants' kidneys show an adult pattern of echoes by four months of age.

A Aetiology of increased cortical echogenicity in neonatal kidneys

   Glomeruli occupy a greater percentage of renal cortex. (18 % in neonates, 8.6 % in adults.)
   There is a greater proportion of cellular component in the glomerular tuft in neonates than adults.
   Twenty per cent of loops of Henle lie in the cortex in the neonate rather than in the medulla.
   Metanephric mesenchyme persists in the renal cortex for the first six months of life.

The renal pyramids should remain hypoechoic relative to the renal cortex regardless of age.

   When a renal parenchymal abnormality is identified it should be assessed with regards to:

   Distribution – Unilateral/bilateral
                  Focal/diffuse
                  Affecting cortex/medulla/both
                  ± loss of corticomedullary
                        differentiation

Renal size
Perirenal/distant anomalies

4.2 ABSENT KIDNEY ON INTRAVENOUS UROGRAPHY

No kidney found on sonography
Renal aplasia
Renal ectopia
Small scarred kidney e.g. infection,
trauma, calculi etc
Liquid pattern in the renal bed
Hydronephrosis
Polycystic disease
Rarely necrotic tumour
Solid kidney identified
a) small: severe renal scarring e.g.
chronic pyelonephritis
renal ischaemia
b) normal   recent ischaemia
size: nephritis
acute obstruction with
minimal collecting system
dilatation
c) large: tumour
renal vein thrombosis
acute obstruction with
minimal collecting system
dilatation

4.2.1 Non-visualized kidney on ultrasonography

When a kidney is absent bowel may lie in the renal bed and may mimic a renal abscess or hydronephrosis.

The adrenal is relatively large in the neonate and be mistaken for a small kidney if the kidney is absent.

> Renal agenesis. Unilateral agenesis affects 1 in 1000 of the population. The contralateral kidney is usually hypertrophied
>
> Renal ectopia
>
> Small kidney – may be difficult to visualize particularly if the parenchyma is echogenic
>
> Displaced kidney – the kidney may be displaced and distorted by an adjacent soft tissue mass
>
> Replaced kidney – the renal parenchyma is replaced by an infiltrative process e.g. neoplasia or xanthogranulomatous pyelonephritis
>
> Horse-shoe kidney – often low in the abdomen and obscured by bowel loops
>
> Pancake kidney – a flat kidney in the lower abdomen. Deformity is due to lack of normal pressure from adjacent structures *in utero*
>
> Hydronephrotic sac – may be mistaken for fluid filled bowel loops
>
> Calcified kidney – e.g. tuberculous auto-nephrectomy
>
> Juxta-renal fluid. Acoustic enhancement due to adjacent fluid may make the kidney difficult to recognize

4.2.2 Renal parenchymal disease

The appearances of the renal parenchyma are normally compared with adjacent structures e.g. hepatic and splenic parenchyma. Adjacent abnormalities such as ascites or hepatic parenchymal disease may make it difficult to evaluate the kidney. Also, even with histological and clinical evidence of renal parenchymal disease the kidney may appear normal particularly in the acute stage of disease.

A Classification of the renal parenchymal echopattern

Grade	Appearance
0	Normal
1	Parenchymal echogenicity is increased approximately the same as hepatic echogenicity
2	Echogenicity is greater than hepatic parenchyma but less than central echo complex
3	Echogenicity equal to that of the central echocomplex

There is no correlation between the degree of parenchymal echogenicity and the nature of the underlying disease process though the degree of echogenicity is roughly related to the degree of sclerosis, fibrosis, tubular atrophy and cellular infiltrate.

B Classification of renal parenchymal disease

Distribution of sonographic abnormality:

Type 1   Accentuated cortical echoes
Renal pyramids remain normal with normal cortico-medullary differentiation

Type 2   Generalized parenchymal abnormality with loss of cortico-medullary differentiation.

In the early stages of medical renal disease the kidneys are typically enlarged. In the late stages they are small and usually echogenic with loss of corticomedullary differentiation whatever the disease and initial sonographic appearances. Thus a kidney initially showing type 1 changes may progress to type 2 changes later in the disease.

4.3 CAUSES OF TYPE 1 CHANGES

Acute glomerulonephritis
Chronic glomerulonephritis
Lupus nephritis
Lipoid nephrosis
Hypersensitivity angiitis
Acute/chronic transplant rejection
Bilateral renal vein thrombosis
Alport's disease
Leukaemia (the only malignancy causing type 1 changes.)
Nephrosclerosis (hypertension/diabetes)
Tubular nephritis
Amyloid
Acute tubular necrosis
Beckwith Wiedemann syndrome
Myeloglobinuric renal failure
Kawasaki disease
Cortical nephrocalcinosis
AIDS
Early polycystic disease
Tutular necrosis

4.4 CAUSES OF TYPE 2 CHANGES

(Focal or diffuse disruption of parenchymal anatomy with loss of cortico-medullary differentiation.)
Acute bacterial nephritis (lobar nephronia)
Chronic pyelonephritis
Chronic glomerulonephritis
Healing infarcts
Infantile polycystic disease
Adult polycystic disease
Glomerular polycystic disease
Medullary cystic disease
Many of the causes of type 1 changes result in type 2 parenchymal changes with small echogenic kidneys with lack of cortico-medullary differentiation in the late stages.

4.4.1 Acute nephritis

Acute glomerulonephritis is usually due to the presence of circulating immune complexes or autoimmune disease which cause renal damage. The main use of sonography in these patients who may present with rapidly failing renal function is to exclude hydronephrosis and surgically treatable causes of renal failure. Initially the kidney appears normal or enlarged. As the disease progresses the renal parenchyma becomes echogenic though less often oedema causes a reduction in parenchymal echogenicity. (In children renal oedema may cause increased parenchymal echogenicity due to disruption of tissue interfaces.)

4.4.2 Chronic pyelonephritis

In longstanding cases the renal size returns to normal and then shrinks resulting in bilateral small contracted echogenic kidneys.

4.4.3 Nephrosclerosis

This is usually the end result of prolonged hypertension. The kidney may appear normal or small with echogenic parenchyma.

4.5 NEONATAL KIDNEY – DIFFUSE INCREASE IN ECHOGENICITY

Normal
Infantile polycystic disease
Renal vein thrombosis
Cortical nephrocalcinosis
Early stages of adult polycystic disease
Glomerulocystic disease
Congenital/neonatal nephrotic syndrome

4.6 UNILATERAL SMALL KIDNEY

Ischaemia
Post obstructive atrophy
Unilateral chronic pyelonephritis/reflux
Radiation nephritis
Renal tuberculosis
Congenital hypoplasia
Post traumatic atrophy
Heminephrectomy

4.7 BILATERAL SMALL KIDNEYS

Old age
Nephrosclerosis
Ischaemic atrophy
Chronic pyelonephritis/reflux
Chronic glomerulonephritis
Bilateral obstructive/postobstructive atrophy
Papillary necrosis (late)
Bilateral infarction (late)
Arteritis e.g. polyarteritis nodosa
Hereditary nephritis
Medullary cystic disease
Scleroderma (late)
Renal cortical necrosis
Gout nephropathy
Chronic lead poisoning
Hypertensive nephropathy
Diabetic nephropathy
Hyperparathyroidism (late)
Any longstanding renal parenchymal disease
    may result in bilateral small kidneys

4.7.1 Renal fibrolipomatosis

The presence of excess fat in the renal sinus enlarges the central echocomplex so that the renal parenchymal tissue appears relatively narrow. Rarely the enlarged central echocomplex is anechoic but usually the excess fat is of high echogenicity. The fatty nature of the tissue in the renal sinus may be confirmed by computerized tomography. When the renal sinus fat is hypoechoic the appearances may be mistaken for parapelvic cysts, hydronephrosis or transitional cell carcinoma.

4.7.2 Renal oedema

Renal oedema usually causes a reduction in renal echogenicity. This is particularly prominent in the renal pyramids which may appear anechoic and may be mistaken for cysts. The renal capsule may also appear unusually prominent. Less commonly renal oedema causes a transient increase in parenchymal echogenicity due to disruption of tissue interfaces.

A Aetiology of oedema

Acute glomerulonephritis
Acute pyelonephritis
Nephrotic syndrome
Transplant rejection
Renal contusion

4.8 ECHOGENIC FOCUS WITH THINNING OF OVERLYING PARENCHYMA

Normal variant
Focal infarct
Pyelonephritic scar
Tuberculous scar
Renal papillary necrosis

4.8.1 Renal calcification

Small calcific foci are seen as very echogenic foci. As these foci enlarge they cause distal acoustic shadowing. When the kidney is densely calcified it may be difficult to recognize and may be indistinguishable from gas-filled bowel loops.

A Renal parenchymal calcification

Medullary calcification
Cortical calcification
Calcification in a cyst wall – usually a complicated cyst. Three per cent of renal cysts show wall calcification.
Calcification in a renal tumour – usually amorphous but can be ring-like and mimic cyst wall calcification. Calcification is seen in 6 % of tumours.

4.8.2 Medullary calcinosis

Medullary nephrocalcinosis may occur in any case of hypercalcaemia or hypercalcuria. It gives rise to densely echogenic medullary pyramids which may cause shadowing. This may be evident on ultrasonography before it is seen on abdominal radiography.

A   Aetiology

Hyperparathyroidism
Milk-alkali syndrome
Renal tubular acidosis (distal type)
Extensive malignancy ± bone involvement
Vitamin D excess
Idiopathic hypercalcuria
Idiopathic hypercalcaemia of infancy
Cushing's disease/syndrome
Prolonged bed rest, particularly with underlying
    bone disease
Medullary sponge kidney
Frusemide therapy in preterm infants
Sarcoidosis

4.9   DIFFERENTIAL DIAGNOSIS OF ECHNOGENIC RENAL PYRAMIDS

Calcification
Renal tubular ectasia disorders –
          Infantile polycystic kidneys
          Juvenile polycystic kidneys
Renal pyramidal fibrosis – usually forms part
    of a generalized parenchymal abnormality

4.9.1   Renal cortical calcification

Renal cortical calcification causes increased cortical echogenicity with complete shadowing in severe cases. Secondary pyramidal fibrosis may occur.

A Aetiology

Chronic glomerulonephritis
Renal cortical necrosis
Alport's disease
Acute transplant rejection
Oxalosis – may cause medullary calcinosis or both
cortical and medullary calcification

B Nephrocalcinosis and nephrolithiasis in children

64 % are associated with an underlying structural
renal lesion or urinary tract infection
10 % are associated with hypercalcaemia or hypercalcuria
6 % are associated with cystinuria
20 % — idiopathic (up to 50 % in some series),
oxalosis and miscellaneous conditions

4.9.2 Renal emphysema

Renal emphysema is gas in or around the kidney. It
causes densely echogenic areas with distal shadowing.

A Aetiology

Surgery
Instrumentation
Infections with gas forming organisms (particularly
in diabetics)
Fistula with bowel

B Main differential diagnosis

calculi
renal calcification

4.9.3 Xanthogranulomatous pyelonephritis

This is a chronic inflammatory condition usually secondary to chronic infection (e.g. *Proteus* and *E. coli*) and

renal calculi. The kidney is replaced by sheets of inflammatory and 'foam' cells. Diagnosis is difficult and sonographic, urographic and angiographic findings may all mimic tumour. Sonography shows an enlarged and relatively sonolucent kidney. Calculi are frequently present but are often difficult to identify. The kidney may be generally hypoechoic or it may show echogenic and hypoechoic foci.

4.9.4 Malakoplakia

This is also an uncommon inflammatory renal disorder. The kidney is enlarged and may show a normal echotexture, a nodular pattern, cyst-like areas or loss of differentiation between the parenchyma and central echocomplex echoes.

4.9.5 AIDS nephropathy

Renal disease in AIDS is an important cause of mortality and morbidity. It is associated with almost a 100 % mortality within six months of the onset of uraemia despite the use of dialysis. The following pathological changes have been reported:

    Segmental glomerulosclerosis
    Interstitial fibrosis
    Mononuclear cell infiltrate
    Interstitial nephritis
    Dilated tubules containing hyaline casts
    Tubular atrophy
    Acute tubular necrosis
    Focal nephrocalcinosis

These pathological changes may also occur in heroin associated nephropathy. Renal infections are common and result in variable proteinuria and renal insufficiency. Sonography may show extensive parenchymal abnormality usually associated with increased parenchymal echogenicity.

4.10 NEPHROMEGALY WITH A NORMAL ECHOTEXTURE

Acute processes:
>   Acute pyelonephritis
>   Interstitial nephritis
>   Renal tubular necrosis
>   Renal vein thrombosis

Chronic processes:
>   Compensatory hypertrophy
>   Amyloid
>   Leukaemic infiltration
>   Lymphoma (diffuse infiltration or reactive changes)
>   Metastatic infiltration
>   Malakoplakia (75 % of cases show multifocal changes but 25 % show diffuse disease which may not be detectable)

4.11 UNILATERAL RENAL ENLARGEMENT

Normal variant e.g. duplex collecting system
Duplication
Pyelonephritis
Hypertrophy due to contralateral renal disease
Hydronephrosis
Neoplasia. Primary or secondary
Renal vein thrombosis
Cystic disease
Multicystic renal dysplasia
Pyonephrosis
Xanthogranulomatous pyelonephritis
Malakoplakia

4.12 FOCAL RENAL ENLARGEMENT

Primary or secondary malignancy
Cyst
Abscess
Acute lobar nephritis/acute lobar nephronia
Enlarged septum of Bertin
Dromedary hump
Haematoma
Renal lobe supplied by an aberrant artery
Focal xanthogranulomatous pyelonephritis or
    malakoplakia
Pseudomass lesion

4.13 BILATERAL RENAL ENLARGEMENT

Multiple simple cysts
Polycystic disease
Bilateral duplex kidneys
Bilateral obstruction/hydronephrosis
Acute glomerulonephritis
Nephrotic syndrome
Diabetic nephropathy
Amyloid
Surgery
Leukaemia
Lymphoma
Bilateral renal neoplasms. Primary or
  secondary
Gaucher's disease
Tuberous sclerosis with hamartomas
Acute arteritis
Acromegaly
Myeloma
Bilateral renal vein thrombosis
Acute tubular necrosis
Acute uric acid nephropathy
Total parenteral nutrition
Renal lymphangioma
Nephroblastomatosis
Beckwith–Wiedemann syndrome
Xanthogranulomatous pyelonephritis

4.13.1 Renal vascular disease

A *Renal vein thrombosis*
This uncommon condition occurs most frequently in
neonates usually secondary to dehydration caused by

diarrhoea, vomiting or sepsis. It is also associated with the nephrotic syndrome, glomerulonephritis, tumour, trauma and pregnancy. In adults tumour extension into the renal vein is the commonest cause. The left renal vein is affected three times more frequently than the right as it is longer and is compressed between the aorta and superior mesenteric artery. Thrombosis begins in the arcuate and interlobular veins and extends to the renal veins hence most cases are unilateral. Intravenous urography shows impaired renal function with a delayed and prolonged nephrogram. On ultrasonography the kidney is initially enlarged with reduced cortical echogenicity. Haemorrhage may distort the central sinus echoes. In the subacute stage (7–14 days) the cortex becomes echogenic with preservation of cortico-medullary differentiation due to cellular infiltration. Hypoechoic areas may persist due to focal haemorrhage. Thrombus may be visible within the renal vein as intraluminal echoes and Doppler scanning shows reduced or absent flow. Development of collateral venous drainage may allow the kidney to return to normal or it may atrophy producing a small echogenic kidney in which corticomedullary differentiation may be preserved or lost.

B Renal artery thrombosis

Renal artery thrombosis is rare in children and is usually secondary to dehydration, maternal diabetes, umbilical artery catheters or emboli via a patent ductus arteriosus. In adults it is usually secondary to severe atheroma, trauma, arteritis, aneurysm or fibromuscular hyperplasia. If visualized the artery shows internal echoes with decreased or absent flow on Doppler studies. Focal infarction may give rise to echogenic or hypoechoic areas which may have a mass effect. Echogenic infarcts usually become hypoechoic over a few days. Eventually the infarct atrophies causing parenchymal thinning. If the whole kidney is ischaemic it may appear normal or enlarged but becomes hypoechoic and then atrophies giving rise to a small scarred kidney. Renal artery trauma gives rise to similar appearances and although Doppler studies can confirm reduced or absent arterial flow a normal ultrasound scan does not exclude renal artery damage or thrombosis.

C Renal cortical necrosis
This unusual condition occurs more frequently in children than in adults. It occurs due to severe hypotension or hypoxia which is usually secondary to dehydration, sepsis, blood loss, hypoxia, haemoglobinopathy or the haemolytic/uraemic syndrome. In the acute stage the kidney is normal in size or enlarged. There is a subcapsular rim of reduced echogenicity. In subacute and longstanding cases this area of cortex becomes echogenic and may calcify. Secondary medullary fibrosis may also occur.

D Acute tubular necrosis
Acute tubular (medullary) necrosis occurs secondary to severe compromise to renal perfusion or hypoxia. Sonographic appearances are variable as tubules are found both in the medulla and the renal cortex. The kidney frequently appears normal. Other findings include variable increase in the pyramidal echogenicity though the renal pyramids usually remain well defined. Increased pyramidal echogenicity may be associated with variable increase in cortical echogenicity. The renal pyramids may appear swollen and this may

give the central echo complex a scalloped outline. Uncommonly the pyramids are of reduced echogenicity.

E Renal trauma
Renal trauma is common in both adults and children and ultrasonography is valuable in detecting many of the complications of trauma such as renal haematomas, lacerations and contusions. Though Doppler studies may confirm arterial flow they cannot exclude arterial damage and intravenous urography, isotope studies or angiography may be necessary to confirm perfusion and function. When assessing the kidney in trauma cases adjacent organs should also be evaluated as renal damage may be associated with hepatic or splenic injury. In cases of trauma renal damage is more likely if there is an underlying renal pathology such as hydronephrosis.

F Renal contusion
Appearances are variable depending upon the state of the blood in the contusion/haematoma. Initially blood is hypoechoic but it rapidly becomes echogenic as it clots. Later the haematoma liquifies and the collection becomes hypoechoic, anechoic or complex. The contusion may be seen as a defect in the renal contour.

G Renal haematoma
Subcapsular haematomas spread around the kidney giving rise to an echogenic rim. Focal subcapsular haematomas may depress the cortex. As the haematoma resolves fibrosis may occur which may compress the kidney resulting in hypertension. Intra-renal haematomas are more frequently hypoechoic than renal contusions and subcapsular haematomas. Echogenic

haematomas may be lost in the central echocomplex. Renal haematomas may enlarge and thus they should be followed up as they may cause delayed rupture of the kidney.

H Peri-renal haematoma

These haematomas initially appear anechoic but rapidly become moderately echogenic. Peri-renal haematomas do not usually change the renal shape but may expand into the anterior or posterior pararenal spaces. Large collections may appear septate and may contain both blood and urine.

4.14 RENAL FAILURE

Renal failure is a degree of renal insufficiency which causes substantial alteration in plasma biochemistry. The main uses of ultrasonography in renal failure are the exclusion of obstruction to urine drainage, demonstration of renal parenchymal abnormalities and guided biopsy. Acute renal failure is due to obstruction to drainage in only 5 % of cases. Sonography can reliably exclude dilatation of the urinary tract but this does not entirely exclude obstruction particularly if the patient is dehydrated and in cases of doubt antegrade pyelography should be performed. Polyuric renal failure may cause distension of the urinary tract particularly if the patient is scanned with a full bladder and this may be mistaken for obstruction.

4.15 CAUSES OF RENAL FAILURE

Poor perfusion – Pre-renal renal failure
  Major vessel disease e.g.
    renal artery avulsion
    renal artery embolus
  Congestion – renal vein thrombosis
Renal disease – Acute tubular necrosis
  Acute glomerulonephritis
  Interstitial nephritis
  Small vessel disease e.g.
    malignant hypertension
    haemolytic–uraemic synd.
  Multiple renal infarcts
  Polycystic disease
  Infection
  Metabolic disorders e.g.
    diabetes
    amyloid
    gout
    dysproteinaemia
  Radiation nephritis
  Renal tubular disease e.g. tubular
    acidosis
Urinary tract obstruction – Bladder
  outflow obstruction e.g. prostatism
  Bilateral ureteric obstruction.

4.15.1 Myoglobinuria

Myoglobinuria occurs when muscle necrosis allows myoglobin to enter the blood stream. Severe cases cause acute renal failure. Sonographically the kidneys appear swollen with increased cortical echogenicity with preservation of the corticomedullary junction.

4.15.2 The transplanted kidney

The transplanted kidney is usually situated in the iliac fossa on the opposite side from which it was derived. It is superficial and thus accessible to examination with high frequency probes. A baseline scan is often taken around five days post transplant to assess renal size, shape, volume and echopattern. Immediately after the operation the kidney appears normal. It then becomes oedematous making the pyramids appear sonolucent relative to the central sinus. There is frequently slight fullness of the collecting system which should not be assumed to be due to obstruction. After transplantation the kidney hypertrophies, renal volume increasing by around 22 % by the end of the third week. A greater increase in renal volume suggests rejection.

N.B. In the transplanted kidney the renal pelvis is usually anterior with the renal artery and vein lying posteriorly.

4.15.3 Acute rejection

Rejection is a dynamic process and not an all or nothing phenomenon. It may be affected by many factors particularly the administration of drugs. This results in a wide spectrum of disease severity which in turn gives a spectrum of sonographic changes. Initially the kidney becomes swollen with large sonolucent pyramids increasing corticomedullary differentiation. Conversely renal parenchyma can also be sonolucent reducing corticomedullary differentiation.

$$\frac{\text{renal pyramid length} \times \text{pyramid width}}{\text{cortical thickness}} = 4.6$$

During acute rejection renal pyramidal swelling increases this index to around 7.5.

Rejection may cause reduced echogenicity of the central echocomplex which may eventually be reduced to a small group of echogenic foci. Areas of haemorrhage and infarction may give rise to a heterogenous echopattern. The wall of the renal pelvis may become oedematous and renal swelling causes increase in the renal volume. When renal volume increases suddenly or severely the renal transplant may actually rupture spontaneously.

Renal volume is approximately equal to renal length × width × depth × 0.49. It normally increases by 16 % (7–25 %) in the first two weeks after transplantation and by 22 % (14–32 %) in the first three weeks.

A Signs of rejection

Increased renal volume
>20 % in   5 days
>25 % in 14 days
>30 % in 21 days
Decreased amplitude of central sinus echoes
Enlarged and abnormally echolucent pyramids
High level echoes in the cortex
Heterogenous echopattern due to areas of haemorrhage and infarction
Renal swelling and haematoma
Renal rupture
Renal vein thrombosis with global swelling
Submucosal swelling of the collecting system
Perinephric fluid (non-specific)
Doppler changes – Decreased diastolic flow
Increased pulstility of the waveform

(The pyramids may appear large and hypoechoic during

a diuresis and in acute tubular necrosis. Increased renal volume may occur in renal vein thrombosis, pyelonephritis and cytomegalovirus infection.)

4.15.4 Chronic rejection

Initially the kidney is of normal size but cortical echogenicity increases due to periglomerular cellular infiltration and cortical fibrosis. The kidney slowly reduces in size and the pyramids become increasingly echogenic causing loss of corticomedullary differentiation. Appearances are eventually the same as any end stage renal parenchymal disease.

4.16 ACUTE POST-TRANSPLANTATION RENAL FAILURE

Acute tubular necrosis
Acute rejection
Arterial obstruction
Renal vein thrombosis
Ureteric obstruction
Pyelonephritis
Cytomegalovirus infection

4.17 TRANSPLANT HYDRONEPHROSIS

4.17.1 Aetiology

(Slight collecting system dilatation is normal)

Ureteric oedema
Ureteric stricture
Ureteric ischaemia
Extrinsic compression – lymphocoele
                              haematoma
                              urinoma
                              abscess
Calculi
Clot in the collecting system or ureter

4.17.2 Fluid collection around a transplanted kidney

A thin rim of fluid around a transplanted kidney is a common finding and should not be assumed to be pathological.

Haematoma. May be post operative or due to complications such as rejection, ischaemia, hypertension or biopsy

Urinomas are found in 3–10 % of transplants and can cause loss of a kidney. Leakage usually occurs at the anastomosis at the vesicoureteric junction. Late urinomas may be due to biopsy, trauma, infection or ischaemia

Abscess

Lymphocoele. These form in up to 20 % of transplants due to division of lymphatics at surgery. The kidneys produce as much lymph each day as they do urine (1.5–2.0 l) thus the occurrence of lymphocoeles is not surprising. They usually present 2–6 weeks post operation but may be exacerbated by rejection. Eighty per cent show septae and they may compress adjacent vascular structures and the bladder. Sonographic appearances of these fluid collections are non-specific and fine needle aspiration may be necessary for diagnosis.

4.18 RENAL CYSTIC DISEASE

Renal cysts are common incidental findings on ultrasonography but may also form part of a specific disease process. Differentiation of the patterns of cystic disease is necessary for diagnosis.

4.18.1 Classification of renal cystic disease.

A *Renal dysplasia*
> Multicystic dysplastic kidney (Potter 2)
> Focal and segmental dysplasia
> Multiple cysts associated with lower tract obstruction

B *Polycystic disease*
> Autosomal recessive (Potter 1)
> Autosomal dominant (Potter 3)
> Glomerulocystic disease

C *Cortical cysts*
> e.g. Tuberous sclerosis
> Trisomy syndromes 13–15, 17–18
> Potter type 4 – small cortical cyst with obstructive hydronephrosis
> Multilocular cysts
> Chronic dialysis

D *Medullary cysts*

>   Medullary sponge kidney
>   Medullary cystic disease
>   Medullary necrosis
>   Pyelogenic cyst

E *Miscellaneous*

>   Inflammatory cysts
>   Tuberculosis
>   *Echinococcus*
>   Calculus disease
>   Neoplasia – benign cystic nephroma
>   polycystic nephroma

F *Extraparenchymal cysts*

>   Parapelvic – outside renal capsule but
>   adjacent to renal pelvis
>   Perinephric

4.18.3 Adult polycystic disease

Adult polycystic disease is transmitted as an autosomal
dominant condition which affects approximately 1 in
1000 of the population. Presentation is usually with
hypertension and progressive renal failure after the
third decade. Uncommonly it presents in children and
has been seen rarely in neonates. Thirty to forty per
cent of cases are associated with hepatic cysts, 10 %
with pancreatic cysts, 5 % with splenic cysts and
uncommonly pulmonary cysts also occur. These extra-
renal manifestations are not usually found in cases in
neonates and young children. The cysts may arise from
any part of the nephron and occasionally arise from

the glomerulus. They occur as saccular eventrations which enlarge to form cysts.

Ultrasonography is a valuable screening test in cases of suspected polycystic disease. In the early stages of autosomal dominant polycystic disease the cysts may be between 0.1 and 5 mm in diameter. In these cases small cysts may be too small to be visualized sonographically but disruption of renal parenchymal architecture results in increased echogenicity due to the increased number of tissue interfaces. At this stage appearances are indistinguishable from infantile polycystic or glomerulocystic disease though the patient is usually older than patients with the latter two diseases. As the cysts enlarge the sonographic appearances become more typical with enlarged kidneys containing multiple cysts of varying sizes resulting in an irregular renal contour. The cysts may have irregular walls and may show internal echoes if they have been complicated by haemorrhage or infection. Surviving islands of renal parenchyma may be seen between the cysts. When screening for evidence of autosomal dominant polycystic disease if the kidney shows no evidence of cysts or parenchymal abnormality by the age of 19 years the patient is extremely unlikely to be affected.

A Differential diagnosis

Any cause of multiple intrarenal fluid collections
Hydrocalycosis, particularly if the renal pelvis is not dilated
Multiple hypo/anechoic nodules e.g. lymphoma

4.18.4 Autosomal recessive polycystic kidney disease (Infantile polycystic disease)

Infantile polycystic kidney disease is an autosomal recessive condition which usually presents in infancy or childhood though it may be diagnosed *in utero* by ultrasonography. Disease severity is usually greater in cases which present early. There is an association with hepatic periportal fibrosis and ductal hyperplasia which may cause portal hypertension.

The disease may be sub-divided by age at presentation:

> Perinatal form – Presents in babies, rapidly fatal, 90 % of renal tubules are involved
> Infantile form – 60 % of tubules involved, the child is uraemic but survives longer than those with the perinatal form
> Young children – Presentation with hypertension and chronic renal failure. Twenty-five per cent of tubules are involved
> Late presentation (Juvenile form) – Symptoms are usually related to hepatic fibrosis, portal hypertension and gastro-intestinal haemorrhage. In these late cases small cysts can sometimes be seen in the renal cortex

A Sonographic features

The kidneys are smoothly enlarged with multiple small cysts (1–2 mm diameter) which arise from the collecting ducts as fusiform dilatations. The cysts are arranged radially and become more spherical as they enlarge. This diffuse tubular ectasia disrupts renal architecture causing increased parenchymal echogenicity with loss of corticomedullary differentiation. There may be a thin rim of compressed renal parenchyma around the kidney which is hypoechoic relative to the remaining parenchyma which is abnormally echogenic. *In utero* the normal combined renal circumference is 27–30 % of abdominal circumference. In infantile polycystic disease this increases to 60 % allowing prenatal diagnosis.

4.18.5 Glomerulocystic disease

Cysts occur in all parts of the nephron but predominate in the glomerulus. They are usually 2–3 mm in diameter but may be up to 1 cm in diameter and rarely even larger. The majority of visible cysts occur in the cortex and they may be accompanied by interstitial renal disease. Glomerulocystic disease does not usually show Mendelian inheritance but may occur in association with tuberous sclerosis, trisomy 13, the cerebro-hepato-renal syndrome of Zellweger, short ribbed polydactyly syndrome, oro-facio-digital syndrome or renal retinal dysplasia. Generally renal failure occurs early and prognosis is poor.

Sonographic appearances are of enlarged kidneys with very echogenic parenchyma, particularly cortex and occasional small cortical cysts. If no cysts are seen appearances cannot be differentiated from autosomal recessive polycystic disease or early autosomal dominant polycystic disease. If cysts are visible in an echogenic infantile kidney then glomerulocystic disease is more likely than infantile polycystic disease.

4.18.6 Multicystic dysplastic kidney

This is a relatively rare condition but even so it is the commonest cause of an abdominal mass in a neonate.

It occurs due to obstruction to drainage *in utero* and is asssociated with an atretic ureter, small renal artery and there is usually no identifiable collecting system. The underlying obstruction usually occurs at or before 8–10 weeks of life. Obstruction occurring at a later stage gives a combination of renal dysplasia and hydronephrosis.

Sonographic appearances are of a large unilateral renal mass with multiple cysts of differing sizes. There may be islands of dysplastic renal tissue between the cysts but no normal renal tissue is seen.

The contralateral kidney has an increased risk of obstruction to drainage and it should be followed up carefully.

4.19 DIFFERENTIAL DIAGNOSIS OF MULTICYSTIC DYSPLASTIC KIDNEY

Gross hydronephrosis
Multilocular cyst
Cystic nephroma
Cystic hamartoma
Cystic lymphangioma
Perlman tumour
Multiple simple cysts (very rare in children)

If multicystic dysplastic kidney is missed in the neonatal period it will atrophy as it is non-functioning and the cysts calcify.

4.19.1 Medullary cystic disease

Medullary cystic disease forms a spectrum of disease ranging from the relatively benign medullary sponge kidney to the severe juvenile nephronophthosis.

4.19.2 Medullary sponge kidney

This is an uncommon condition in which there is cystic dilatation of the collecting tubules. Though the condition is not familial it appears to be congenital. Presentation usually occurs in the second to fourth decades with abdominal pain, haematuria and pyelonephritis. Thirty per cent of patients also have hypercalcuria and small calculi usually form in the ectatic tubules. The condition is of variable severity and may affect a single lobe of one kidney or it may be found throughout both kidneys. Sonographically the kidneys may appear normal or may show increased pyramidal echogenicity due to the presence of multiple small calculi. Rarely very small cysts are seen.

4.19.3 Juvenile nephronophthosis

Juvenile nephronophthosis is a severe medullary cystic disease which is usually transmitted as an autosomal recessive condition. Presentation is usually in older children or young adults who show severe renal impairment with hypertension, proteinuria and occasionally salt loosing nephropathy. Sonographically the kidneys are normal sized or small with abnormally echogenic parenchyma associated with loss of corticomedullary differentiation. Very small cysts are sometimes seen in the medullary and cortico-medullary areas.

4.19.4 Renal cysts in dialysis

Renal cysts occur in patients in renal failure on long term dialysis. The risk of developing cysts increases with time and eventually 70 % of long term dialysis patients are affected. The cysts are seen in small kidneys with severe parenchymal changes. They are prone to complications such as haemorrhage and are associated with an increased risk of renal carcinoma.

4.19.5　Simple renal cysts

The exact aetiology of simple renal cysts is uncertain, they may be retention cysts due to duct obstruction or they may arise in embryonic rests. They are uncommon in children (found in 2–4 % of paediatric postmortems) but occur with increasing frequency with age and are found in 50 % of adults over 50 years. Simple cysts are usually asymptomatic unless complicated by:

> Haemorrhage or infection
> Very large – mass effect
> Arise in a parapelvic position compressing part of the renal collecting system

A　Sonographic features

> The cyst is entirely echofree
> Good sound transmission gives rise to distal acoustic enhancement
> The cyst has a smooth outline without a demonstrable wall

Small cysts may only appear echofree when they are in the focal zone of the ultrasound beam due to the partial volume effect and very small cysts (<3 mm diameter) cannot be identified in the parenchyma. Ultrasonography is more accurate than computed tomography at visualization of internal septae and demonstrating internal cyst morphology. If there is any doubt about the nature of a cyst identified at sonography then a follow up scan or cyst aspiration should be performed. If the appearances are classically those of a simple cyst then no further action need be taken.

SIMPLE RENAL CYST ASPIRATE –

Fluid is straw coloured

Cyst fluid should not contain fat

Cyst fluid LDH level should be less than the serum LDH level taken at the same time

The cyst should not contain blood or altered blood products

N.B. Sonography cannot reliably differentiate simple cysts from those complicated by infection and aspiration may yield pus even though the cyst appeared anechoic.

ATYPICAL CYSTS –

Shape – not entirely circular or irregular margin

Cyst wall

Outline – irregular – may be due to cyst collapse, haemorrhage or infection but elevations and irregularities of a cyst wall may be due to tumour

Cyst wall calcification is uncommon in simple cysts. It also occurs in tumours and does not differentiate benign and malignant cysts

Fluid contents

Internal echoes are usually due to intracyst haemorrhage or less often infection. Tumours rarely undergo sufficient necrosis to mimic simple cysts. Necrotic tumour usually has a complex appearance. Fine internal septations are usually due to previous haemorrhage or infection.

4.20 ATYPICAL CYSTS

Collapsed old benign cysts
Septated benign cysts
Haemorrhagic benign cysts
Cysts with intracystic carcinoma
Infected benign cyst
Echinococcal cyst
Abscess
Cystic nephroma
Necrotic tumour
Tumour in cyst wall
Cystic degeneration in an adenoma
Focal xanthogranulomatous pyelonephritis

4.21 COMPLEX RENAL MASSES (have both cystic and solid elements – exclude reverberation echoes at the near wall)

Renal tumours – Necrotic tumour
             Adenoma – cystic
             degeneration
             Multilocular cystic nephroma
             Wilms tumour
             Clear cell sarcoma
Metastases
Cysts – Infected
        Haemorrhagic
        Multilocular
        Multiple
Abscess
Duplication with obstruction
Multilocular cyst
Echinococcal cyst

Focal xanthogranulomatous pyelonephritis
Haematoma
Haemorrhagic infarct
Pyonephrosis
Polycystic disease – may mimic a cystic mass
   if cysts are grouped together and
   surrounded by surviving parenchyma

4.22 CALCIFIED CYSTS

Simple cyst (rare)
Tumour
Echinococcal cyst
Calcified old multicystic dysplastic kidney
Calcified old abscess

4.23 HAEMORRHAGIC CYSTS

Haemorrhage in a simple cyst
Liquefied haematoma
Focal infection
Focal infarction
Cystic degeneration in a tumour
(appearances are variable and may be
   identical to a simple cyst or may show
   irregular borders and internal echoes)

4.24 LESIONS WHICH MAY MIMIC RENAL CYSTS

Prominent renal pyramids

Intra-renal vascularmal formations e.g. aneurysm, arteriovenous malformations

Haematoma

Abscess

Focal hydronephrosis

Pyonephrosis

Calyceal diverticulum

Tuberculous cavity

Duplication

Necrotic tumour

Urinoma

Lymphoma and hypoechoic masses. (On high gain settings these deposits may show internal echoes and less distal enhancement than cysts)

4.25 INTRA-RENAL FLUID COLLECTIONS

Cysts including polycystic disease
Calyceal dilatation
Calyceal diverticulum
Renal papillary necrosis
Dilated moiety of a duplex kidney
Hydronephrosis
Abscess
Tuberculous cavity
Necrotic carcinoma/metastasis
Echinococcal cyst
Renal artery aneurysm
Haematoma

4.25.1 Urinary tract infections

Urinary tract infections are common in both adults and children and remain a major cause of morbidity with further risk of renal scarring causing hypertension and chronic renal failure. As a safe non-invasive investigation renal sonography is the initial investigation of choice in cases of urinary tract infection.

A Aims of sonography in urinary tract infection

To demonstrate the presence of two kidneys
To exclude underlying abnormality e.g. hydronephrosis
To assess complications such as abscess or scarring

(Intravenous urography and ultrasonography are insensitive detectors of renal scarring showing changes only in the late stages when there is thinning of the renal parenchyma due to atrophy and fibrosis. A kidney with extensive irreversible damage may appear sonographically normal in the acute stage or for some time after infection. DMSA isotope scanning is a more sensitive means of detecting scarring in these cases.)

4.25.2 Acute pyelonephritis

Acute pyelonephritis is a bacterial infection of the renal parenchyma. Ninety per cent of cases occur in women and predisposing conditions include pregnancy, diabetes mellitus, obstructive uropathy, steroids and immunosuppression. The affected kidney is swollen with an inflammatory cell infiltrate and streaks of pus in the parenchyma.

A Urographic findings

The IVU is normal in 76 % of cases
24 % show

> poor renal function
> renal size normal/increased
> mild calyceal dilatation or blunting
> mild ureteric dilatation
> possible underlying abnormality

B Sonographic findings

> The kidney usually appears normal
> Kidney may be enlarged
> Loss of definition of internal anatomy
> Global decrease in echogenicity
> Fluid in dilated calyx/pelvis/ureter

The majority of affected kidneys do not have an underlying abnormality. Also, performing intravenous urography during an acute infection often results in a poor-quality examination and thus ultrasonography has replaced urography as the initial investigation of choice in cases of acute pyelonephritis. Ultrasonography will also demonstrate complications such as perinephric abscess that are not evident on urography.

RENAL SCARRING – Severe infections cause destruction of renal parenchyma leading to atrophy and fibrosis with thinning of the parenchyma and alteration of the echopattern. Sonography and urography only show these changes at a late stage of evolution. Sonography may show scars on the anterior and posterior renal surfaces which are not visible at urography while urography may show calyceal deformity associated with scarring more clearly than sonography. Isotope scanning with DMSA is a much more sensitive means of detecting early renal scarring than urography or sonography.

4.25.3 Chronic pyelonephritis

Chronic pyelonephritis causes areas of increased echogenicity with parenchymal thinning, reduced renal size and calyceal blunting. Similar renal parenchymal changes also occur in hypertension, focal infarction and chronic glomerulonephritis.

4.25.4 Bacterial nephritis

The kidneys are very vascular organs and may be subject to secondary infection during septicaemia resulting in white cell infiltration. This results in increase in renal size with or without increased parenchymal echogenicity and loss of cortico-medullary differentiation.

4.25.5 Vesico-ureteric reflux

Though ultrasonography is not a sensitive detector of vesico-ureteric reflux we perform pre- and post-micturition renal sonography as a routine. This also allows measurement of the residual volume of urine in the bladder after micturition.

A *Sonographic features of reflux*

Transient visualization of the ureters seen during ultrasound examination may be due to reflux or transient ureteric dilatation during the passage of a wave of peristalsis. More prominent reflux may lead to permanent upper tract dilatation but this may be difficult to differentiate from other causes of upper tract dilatation such as obstruction. If the renal collecting system is seen to be dilated but the ureters are not visualized then the appearances may be mistaken for pelvi-ureteric junction obstruction.

Reflux is common in children being found in 25 % of neonates and infants. The incidence decreases with age and the majority of children have ceased to reflux by the age of two years. Bladder wall oedema during lower urinary tract infection may predispose to reflux as do abnormalities of the vesico-ureteric junction such as 'hutch diverticulum' and ectopic ureters. Reflux with upper tract infection may be the presenting signs of bladder outlet obstruction or neurogenic bladder and bladder function should be carefully assessed prior to surgical reimplantation of the ureters as a treatment for reflux.

4.25.6 Focal pyelonephritis (focal lobar nephronia)

Focal lobar nephronia is a focal bacterial infection of the kidney which causes symptoms similar to those of acute pyelonephritis or renal abscess. Sonography shows focal renal abnormality usually in the form of a focal mass. This may be well defined or poorly defined and is usually anechoic or hypoechoic. The mass may distort the collecting system and central echocomplex.

4.25.7 Renal abscess

A renal abscess may give a spectrum of appearances from those of a simple cyst to debris and air filled collection. Main features include:

Initially the affected area has a hypoechoic semi-solid appearance. This may resolve with treatment or progress

A focal primarily cystic collection

Hypoechoic/anechoic

Margins generally irregular

Walls usually thick

Good transmission of sound though less than that of a simple cyst: variable distal acoustic enhancement

Presence/absence of debris

Presence/absence of gas. Gas bubbles give rise to small highly echogenic foci which may shadow

4.25.8 Post-nephrectomy abscess

A post-nephrectomy abscess gives the appearance of a fluid collection in the renal bed though the presence of echogenic microbubbles may give a solid appearance. Identical appearances may occur with fluid-filled bowel loops lying in the renal bed.

4.25.9 Retained surgical swabs

Retained swabs give the appearance of a densely echogenic mass which at high gain settings may show linear folds. Swabs totally soaked in fluid without any gas present may actually give a woven pattern.

4.25.10 Pyonephrosis

Infection in an obstructed or hydronephrotic kidney may lead to an accumulation of pus within the collecting system. Clinically a pyonephrosis may be suspected if a urinary tract infection proves difficult to treat or if the patient suffers recurrent episodes of septicaemia despite antibiotic treatment.

A Sonographic features

Appearances may be identical to uncomplicated hydronephrosis despite the presence of thick pus in the collecting system. If in doubt aspirate under local anaesthesia

There may be debris or dependent echoes in the collecting system

The urine in the collecting system may appear anechoic but distal acoustic enhancement may be markedly reduced

4.26 INFLAMMATORY PSEUDOTUMOURS

Focal lobar nephronia
Chronic pyelonephritis with areas of hypertrophy
Focal xanthogranulomatous pyelonephritis
Renal tuberculosis
Pyonephrosis
Echinococcus multilocularis

4.26.1 Renal hydatid

Hydatid disease occurs due to infection with *Echinococcus granulosus* or *E. multilocularis*. The liver is the most commonly affected organ but the kidney may also be involved. Granulosus infection usually has a cystic appearance which initially is similar to a simple cyst but becomes more complex with time developing endocysts and membranes. Separation of cyst walls may give rise to the 'floating lily' sign of floating septae. A solid mass appearance may also occur which is more common in multilocularis infection than granulosus. Cyst wall calcification results in a densely echogenic shadowing mass.

4.26.2 Renal candida

Severe systemic candida is quite uncommon, it usually occurs in ill, debilitated diabetic patients or those with immune suppression.

A *Sonographic features*

> Renal enlargement
> Multiple micro-abscesses = frequently too small to
>   visualize
> Multiple abscesses may make the kidney echogenic
>   or hypoechoic
> Bezoars of debris and fungus balls

4.26.3 Renal tuberculosis

The vascular nature of the kidneys allow haematological spread of tuberculosis from distant sites, usually lung or bowel. The bacilli are arrested in or around the glomeruli and give rise to multiple caseating granulomatous foci. At this stage the foci are microscopic and the kidney appears normal. The majority of foci heal but some enlarge and spread to the medulla. These may rupture into the calyces giving rise to cavities which communicate with the collecting system. Bacilluria is common during pulmonary tuberculosis but despite this the majority of patients do not develop any symptoms or signs of renal tuberculosis.

A   Sonographic features

The kidneys appear normal in early cases

Abscesses and cavities are seen as hypoechoic and anechoic collections

Large abscesses may distort the renal contour and may mimic tumours and cysts. Fibrosis and scarring may give an appearance identical to chronic pyelonephritis or multiple renal infarcts. Calcification is common in late cases and varies from punctate foci to dense calcification of the whole kidney. (Tuberculus autonephrectomy)

Bladder tuberculosis causes fibrosis and mucosal thickening leading to a thick walled small volume bladder with vesico-ureteric reflux. Large granulomatous lesions in the ureters or bladder wall may mimic transitional cell lesions

4.27   HYDRONEPHROSIS

The renal collecting system forms part of the echogenic central echocomplex and is frequently not identifiable as a separate structure. Visualization of the collecting system depends upon the rate of urine formation and the rate of urine drainage. The latter depends upon system distensibility, ureteric peristalsis, the degree of bladder fullness and other mechanical factors. Slight collecting system dilatation is a common normal finding during a diuresis or when the bladder is quite full. In these cases the dilatation resolves when the bladder is emptied.

Hydronephrosis is simply dilatation of the renal collecting system. This is not always due to obstruction and similarly obstruction does not always cause hydronephrosis. Hydronephrosis is seen as anechoic fluid in the renal collecting system and pelvis separating the central sinus echoes. Longstanding cases may show secondary thinning of the renal parenchyma. Dilated calyces loose their sharp angular margins and become blunted. When the hydronephrosis is marked the entire collecting system is outlined as a series of connected fluid filled channels.

4.28 LESIONS CONFUSED WITH HYDRONEPHROSIS

Central renal cysts
Multicystic kidney
Parapelvic cysts
Lucent renal pyramids
Pancreatic pseudocysts
Sonolucent renal masses e.g. lymphoma
Renal varices
Renal artery aneurysm
Arteriovenous malformation
Calyceal diverticulum
Renal sinus lipomatosis (rare lucent form)
Anterior lumbar meningocoele

4.29 URINARY TRACT OBSTRUCTION: FALSE NEGATIVE EXAMINATION

Acute obstruction, upper tracts are not yet dilated. Increased intracalyceal pressure may drastically reduce glomerular filtration rate

Dehydration

Intermittent obstruction

Ruptured collecting system

Bladder outflow obstruction

Spontaneous decompression of an obstructed system (backflow)

Staghorn calculus – obscures dilated collecting system

Multiple parapelvic cysts with superimposed obstruction

Misinterpretation of hydronephrosis as polycystic disease

Caliectasis – dilated calyces mistaken for prominent renal pyramids

Retroperitoneal fibrosis. The degree of renal failure is far greater than the degree of urinary tract dilatation

Technical factors e.g. obesity, overlying bowel loops

Obstructed moiety in a duplex kidney – may be atrophic and difficult to visualize

4.30 FALSE POSITIVE DIAGNOSIS OF URINARY TRACT OBSTRUCTION

Normal variants
  Distensible collecting system
  Prominent renal collecting system
  Lucent pyramids
  Congenital megacalyces
  Calyceal diverticula
  Upper tract distension due to a full
    bladder
Upper tract distension
  Diuresis – Overhydration
              Osmotic load
                Diuretics
                Contrast media
                Diabetes insipidus
                Non-oliguric renal failure
Renal cysts mistaken for collecting system
  dilatation
Lesions confused with hydronephrosis (see
  above)
Inflammatory disease
  Acute pyelonephritis – generalized collecting
    system dilatation
  Chronic pyelonephritis – calyceal blunting
  Tuberculosis and other cavities
  Papillary necrosis
  Post infective calyceal distortion
Reflux nephropathy
Post obstructive dilatation

4.30.1 Pelvi-ureteric junction obstruction

Pelvi-ureteric junction obstruction is the commonest
obstruction to urinary drainage in the paediatric patient.

There is great variation in disease severity and age at presentation and the obstruction may evolve over a period of time. It may be uni- or bilateral though in bilateral cases the kidneys may be affected at different times. The left kidney is affected slightly more frequently than the right.

A Sonographic features

Dilatation of the renal collecting system and pelvis without ureteric dilatation. In severe cases there may be marked parenchymal thinning till the kidney eventually becomes 'a bag of water'. Pelvi-ureteric junction obstruction may be intermittent and may only occur during the stress of a diuresis thus in uncertain cases repeat the examination after oral fluids ± intravenous diuretics.

N.B. Reflux can coexist with pelvi-ureteric junction obstruction and may cause ureteric dilatation. Urine may reflux into an obstructed pelvis as the obstruction is usually only in the normal direction of flow.

4.30.2 The kidney in pregnancy

The renal collecting systems and ureters may dilate in pregnancy particularly during the third trimester. Dilatation is most marked at 28 weeks and is usually more prominent on the right than on the left. This is associated with an increased risk of urinary tract infection.

4.31 COLLECTING SYSTEM MASSES

Masses are easier to identify in a dilated than a non-dilated collecting system. The mass may be the cause of the dilatation, a secondary effect or an incidental finding.

4.31.1 Calculus pattern

Echogenic mass with/without
   shadowing

> e.g. Calculus
> Tumour with surface calcification
> Gas
> Calcification in adjacent renal artery
> Surgical stent or drain

4.31.2 Soft tissue pattern

> Transitional cell carcinoma
> Squamous cell carcinoma
> Blood clot
> Adenocarcinoma of renal pelvis (rare)
> Pyonephrosis, debris/sludge
> Fungus ball
> Sloughed papilla
> Leukoplakia/cholesteatoma
> Malakoplakia

4.31.3 Renal calculi

Renal calculi give rise to densely echogenic foci with distal shadowing unless they are narrower than the ultrasound beam. Non-shadowing calculi are easily lost in the central echocomplex if the collecting system is not dilated.

4.31.4 Renal tumours

With careful scanning up to 97 % of renal tumours may be demonstrated sonographically though there are many causes of renal masses and biopsy is often required to make a firm diagnosis. In view of the potentially serious consequences of missing a renal malignancy any solid renal mass should initially be assumed to be a tumour until proven otherwise. Computerized tomography and ultrasonography are complimentary in the diagnosis and staging of renal malignancy but if a mass is found on ultrasonography, computerized tomography frequently fails to shorten the differential diagnosis and percutaneous biopsy is usually more rewarding. Should a mass be shown to be malignant then computerized tomography is the most accurate means of staging. Ultrasonography alone is usually reliable at excluding renal masses as a means of screening.

4.31.5 Renal pseudotumours

Renal pseudotumours are real or simulated masses which resemble neoplasms but which are composed of histologically normal renal tissue.

Columnar hypertrophy. Hypertrophy of the column or septum of Bertin gives rise to a projection of cortex between the medullary pyramids which may indent the central echocomplex and simulate a mass. The mass is of the same echogenicity as the cortex. These masses are usually less than

3 cm in diameter, they do not distort the renal contour and show normal uptake of technetium DMSA on isotope scanning.

Marginal infra-splenic hump. The 'dromedary hump' is often seen on the lateral aspect of the left kidney due to splenic impression.

Foetal lobulation. Lobulation of the renal contour corresponds to renal lobular architecture.

Hypertrophy of the renal hilum margin. A pseudo-mass may be seen if the renal hilum is scanned obliquely due to renal tissue protruding over the hilum.

Renal sinus lipomatosis. Central echoes are sparse and echofree areas are seen in the sinus which may be mistaken for masses.

Lobulation due to prominent renal pyramids.

4.31.6 Solid renal masses

A solid renal mass
> Distorts renal architecture
> Has a mass effect
> Absorbs sound
> Usually shows internal echoes
> A very uniform mass may appear anechoic
> A hyperechoic mass is often very vascular
> If far wall echoes are present they are less prominent than with cysts

4.32 A SOLID MASS APPEARANCE MAY OCCUR WITH MASSES OTHER THAN TUMOURS
e.g.

Pseudotumours
Complex cysts
Abscess
Haematoma
Malakoplakia
Xanthogranulomatous pyelonephritis
Infarct
Acute lobar nephronia
Contusion

4.32.1 Renal tumours

Benign tumours. These are usually small and are frequently chance findings e.g.

Adenoma
Myoma
Lipoma
Haemangioma
Fibroma
Angiomyolipoma
Hamartoma
Multilocular cystic nephroma
Mesoblastic nephroma (hamartoma, congenital Wilms tumour)

4.32.2 Malignant tumours

Nearly all clinically significant tumours are malignant. Over 80 % of these are renal cell carcinomas. Others include

Transitional cell tumours
Nephroblastoma/Wilms tumour
Clear cell carcinoma
Sarcoma
Lymphoma
Leukaemia
Metastases (very common post mortem findings)

4.32.3 Renal surveillance

Ultrasonography is of value in long term follow up of patients who have had nephrectomy for carcinoma. It is also of value in the surveillance of patients with a high risk of renal tumours provided it is performed at regular intervals e.g. every two or three months. (If follow up is less frequent a tumour may be at an advanced stage when diagnosed.)

A *Conditions associated with an increased risk of renal neoplasm*

Previous neoplasm
Hemihypertrophy (may present after tumour diagnosis)
Aniridia
Beckwith–Wiedemann syndrome
Tuberous sclerosis
Von Hippel Lindau syndrome
Long term dialysis cases
Polycystic disease

4.33 PAEDIATRIC RENAL MASSES

Cystic
  Hydronephrosis
  Duplication with obstructed moiety
  Multicystic dysplastic kidney
  Adult polycystic disease
  Cystic Wilms tumours
  Multiseptate urinoma
  Multilocular cystic nephroma
  Haematoma
  Abscess
Solid pattern
  Wilms tumour
  Hamartoma
  Nephroblastomatosis
  Mesoblastic nephroma
  Infantile polycystic disease
  Rhabdomyosarcoma
  Leiomyosarcoma
  Angiomyolipoma
  Haemangioma
  Haemangiopericytoma
  Mucosal epithelial tumours
  Clear cell sarcoma
  Renal cell carcinoma
  Metastases
  Lymphoma
  Leukaemia
  Pseudotumours

4.34 ECHOGENIC RENAL MASSES

Renal malignancy
Benign renal tumours e.g.
    Hamartoma
    Angioma
    Angiomyolipoma
Abscess with microbubble formation
Mature hydatid cyst
Haematoma
Renal infarct scar
Partly thrombosed renal artery aneurysm
Previous surgery (defect packed with perirenal fat)
Metastasis (usually echopoor)
Renal sinus lipomatosis, particularly focal cases
Focal renal dysplasia
Juxtaglomerular tumour
Liposarcoma
Oncocytoma
Calcified renal cyst or aneurysm
Complicated cyst

4.35 HYPOECHOIC RENAL MASSES

Renal pseudotumour
Renal malignancy
Metastasis
Acute focal bacterial nephritis
Early abscess
Infarct
Contusion
Haematoma
Lymphoma
Arteriovenous malformation
Benign tumours (exceptional)
Xanthogranulomatous pyelonephritis

4.36 RENAL ENLARGEMENT WITH A HETEROGENOUS ECHOPATTERN

Tumours e.g.
    Renal cell carcinoma
    Wilms tumour
    Sarcoma
    Transitional cell carcinoma
Malakoplakia (nodular form)
Xanthogranulomatous pyelonephritis (nodular
   form)
Multiple abscesses
Leukaemia/lymphoma – focal deposits
Contusion/intra-renal clot

N.B. Most of the causes of an echogenic renal mass may give a heterogenous appearance.

4.36.1 Renal adenocarcinoma

Renal adenocarcinoma is a relatively common malignancy accounting for 90 % of primary renal malignancies. It is a primary epithelial neoplasm which arises from the proximal convoluted tubule. Nearly all cases occur in adults though it has been recorded in children less than 10 years of age. Early cases are seen as small cortical based masses which enlarge and invade the renal parenchyma. Late cases may present with the classic triad of loin pain, flank mass and haematuria. Five per cent of patients have bilateral tumours though these are not usually simultaneous.

A Sonographic features

There is a wide spectrum of appearances depending upon the extent of the tumour. The commonest appearance is of a renal mass of increased echogenicity which corresponds to an area of increased vascularity on angiography. There is no true capsule and the margins of the mass are usually irregular though there may be a pseudocapsule of compressed renal parenchyma. Areas of haemorrhage and necrosis may occur within the tumour giving rise to hypoechoic foci and a generally heterogenous appearance. Six to twenty per cent show evidence of calcification (up to 3 % of renal cysts show calcification – peripheral calcification in cysts and tumours may obscure the true internal echopattern) and punctate calcification within a mass occurs almost exclusively in tumours. Growth of the tumour mass may be rapid or slow but when large the mass may completely replace the kidney. The renal veins, inferior vena cava, para-aortic region, retroperitoneal space, liver and contralateral kidney should be inspected for evidence of tumour spread. (Extension of tumour into the renal vein occurs in 4–30 % of cases.) Tumour within the renal vein causes widening of the vein with internal echoes.

TUMOUR IN THE INFERIOR VENA CAVA e.g. –

Renal malignancy
Phaeochromocytoma
Malignant melanoma
Choriocarcinoma
Angiomyolipoma

4.36.2 Patterns of tumour in the inferior vena cava

Mass with low level echoes within the IVC lumen (The IVC is widened)
Complete IVC thrombosis with collateral vessels
Foci of thrombus and tumour adhering to the IVC wall

A Other patterns of renal tumour

Necrotic tumour. Large tumours, usually over 6 cm in diameter, may show necrotic areas.
Cystic tumour. A true cystic appearance is exceptional. A cystic pattern is more common in cystadenocarcinoma which shows thick and thin septae with solid areas.
Intracystic carcinoma. Tumour within a simple cyst can only be detected as tumour nodules when the nodules are greater than 3 mm in diameter.
Pedunculated tumours. Tumours arising close to the renal surface may protrude and grow in a pedunculated manner.
Subcapsular haematoma. Rarely a small tumour may

present with haemorrhage forming a subcapsular haematoma.

4.36.3 Wilms tumour

Wilms tumour is the commonest renal neoplasm in childhood. Eighty per cent of cases present under five years of age with a mean age at presentation of three years. The tumour usually presents as a rapidly-growing, painless, abdominal mass. Microscopic haematuria, fever and leukocytosis may occur and the blood pressure is elevated in 50 % of cases. Tumours are bilateral in 5–13 % of cases though the second tumour may be a metastasis.

A Sonographic appearances

A large solid mass.

Well circumscribed, the majority do not break through the renal capsule

Echogenicity is variable. Generally echogenic

Necrotic areas may give rise to a heterogenous pattern with hypoechoic/anechoic areas

Calcification is uncommon, it is usually irregular and amorphous

Tumour may spread to renal veins and IVC

Any solid renal mass in a young child should be assumed to be a Wilms tumour till proven otherwise

4.36.4 Renal blastema/nephroblastomatosis/epithelial nephroblastoma

These are inter-related conditions closely related to the Wilms tumour. Islands of renal blastema persist in the newborn kidney though they are rarely seen after four months of age. A small percentage progress to become Wilms tumours and others may form the less malignant epithelial nephroblastoma. Rarely there are sufficient nodules of primitive renal blastema within the kidney to cause enlargement. The kidneys then appear enlarged and lobulated with multiple hypoechoic areas. More frequently this tissue is evident on histology but not seen on sonography.

4.36.5 Epithelial nephroblastoma

Epithelial nephroblastoma or cystic Wilms tumour (multilocular cystic nephroma/polycystic nephroblastoma) is less malignant than Wilms tumour and may appear cystic or papillary. In its very benign form it gives rise to a multilocular cystic renal disease. Ultrasonography and computerized tomography cannot predict the degree of malignancy.

4.36.6 Multilocular cystic nephroma (Multilocular cystic nephroma/cystic adenoma/ Perlman tumour/benign nephroblastoma)

These are rare well encapsulated tumours which occur in young children. They may have a non-specific solid appearance if they contain only small cysts but gain a cystic appearance as the cysts enlarge. These cysts contain multiple frond-like protrusions and they may eventually calcify. Histologically they may contain both benign and malignant tissue. Clinically they are usually benign though post surgery recurrence and metastases have been reported.

4.36.7 Mesoblastic nephroma

Mesoblastic nephroma or congenital Wilms tumour is a benign hamartoma. It is a relatively common tumour in the neonate and young infant. It occurs at a younger age than Wilms tumour but has similar sonographic appearances. The tumour is usually benign but can be malignant and gives rise to a solid renal mass which may be quite large (a large renal mass in a child less than one year in age is more likely to be a mesoblastic nephroma than a Wilms tumour). The tumour has a relatively homogenous pattern of low level echoes though haemorrhage and necrosis can give rise to anechoic areas.

4.36.8 Cystic neoplasms

Cysts with intraluminal or intramural tumour are extremely rare in the kidney. A neoplasm surrounded by and masked by simple renal cysts is more likely. Cysts containing tumour usually show wall irregularity, intraluminal echoes and internal septa.

4.36.9 Pseudocystic tumours

Tumours with extensive haemorrhage or necrosis may show large cyst-like areas. Extensive necrosis is uncommon but may occur in advanced Wilms tumours and less frequently in renal carcinoma or clear cell tumours.

4.36.10 Urothelial carcinoma

Urothelial carcinomas arise from the epithelium lining the collecting system, ureters or bladder. The majority are transitional cell carcinomas, squamous cell tumours are less frequent. The tumour gives rise to a mass of low-level echoes though it may appear quite echogenic when surrounded by urine. Tumour encrustation with calcium salts may also increase echogenicity and cause shadowing. Collecting system tumours give rise to low-level echoes within the central echocomplex and may also cause localized hydronephrosis. Bladder lesions give rise to intraluminal filling defects which are attached to the bladder wall by a broad or narrow base. They may change configuration as the patient moves but they are not truly mobile. Rarely tumour haemorrhage is seen as pinpoint echoes arising from the tumour surface. Advanced transitional cell tumours may show extensive invasion of the kidney causing destruction of normal intrarenal anatomy.

4.36.11 Renal lymphoma

Renal lymphoma is usually associated with disease elsewhere and occurs most frequently in longstanding cases. Forty-one per cent of longstanding cases of non-Hodgkins lymphoma eventually show renal involvement. Primary renal lymphoma is rare. Disease may be uni- or bilateral and may be focal or diffuse.

A *Sonographic features*

Renal enlargement
Focal or diffuse areas of reduced echogenicity
Anechoic areas may mimic cysts but show little or no distal enhancement
Diffuse disease causes loss of corticomedullary differentiation

4.36.12 Renal leukaemia

Renal abnormality is common in childhood leukaemia. Cellular infiltration of the renal interstitium occurs though this is not necessarily by leukaemic cells and may be a secondary inflammatory infiltrate. This results in bilateral renal enlargement. Renal cortex may appear normal or show increased or decreased echogenicity. Renal changes may be associated with hepato-splenomegaly and lymphadenopathy. Similar renal changes may occur in renal vein thrombosis, pyelonephritis, lymphoma and glomerulonephritis.

4.36.13 Oncocytomas

These rare renal adenomas were previously classified with the benign renal tumours but are now considered to be part of the spectrum of renal cell carcinoma but without generalized malignant potential. They have also been called granular cell adenomas and eosinophilic adenomas though the actual existence of oncocytomas as a separate disease entity is disputed by some workers. Sonographically these lesions are seen as solitary well defined moderately echogenic masses. They cannot be reliably differentiated from renal cell carcinoma sonographically.

4.36.14 Renal sarcoma

Sarcomas arise from the renal connective tissue though retroperitoneal sarcomas may invade the kidney. They give rise to heterogenous mass lesions.

A Papillary cystadenocarcinoma

These are uncommon renal malignancies which grow slowly and metastasize late. They have a hypoechoic mass appearance which may show areas of necrosis and haemorrhage.

B Renal metastases

Renal metastases are common in patients with advanced malignancy and are frequent post-mortem findings. Occasionally renal metastases are symptomatic and may present before the primary tumour. Renal metastases occur particularly frequently in advanced cases of carcinoma of the lung, breast or melanoma. Sonographically they give rise to renal masses which are usually cortical. The majority are hypoechoic.

4.37 BENIGN RENAL TUMOURS

Epithelial tumours – Adenomas
Non-epithelial tumours – (single tissue)
    Lymphangioma
    Haemangioma
    Fibroma
    Leiomyoma
    Haemangiopericytoma
Non-epithelial tumours – (multiple tissue
  elements)
    Embryonic tumour
    Teratoma
    Angiomyolipoma
    Multilocular cyst
    Cystadenoma
    Tumoral dysplasia

Benign renal tumours are usually well defined round echogenic structures. Only 4 % of renal carcinomas are markedly echogenic and therefore a small echogenic mass is likely to be benign. (As malignancy cannot be excluded all masses which do not contain fat on computerized tomography should be removed.) Adenomas are benign lesions arising from the renal tubules. They may appear hypoechoic.

4.37.1 Haemangioma

Haemangiomas (benign cystic cystadenoma or cystic hamartoma) have a multilocular appearance though careful scanning will show solid intracystic areas.

4.37.2 Arteriovenous malformations

Arteriovenous malformations are frequently too small to visualize though small lesions may still cause significant haemorrhage. When visible they are seen as small hypoechoic lesions. The renal artery and renal vein may be enlarged.

4.37.3 Angiomyolipoma

These are relatively benign mesodermal tumours containing muscle, blood vessels and fat. They may be associated with tuberous sclerosis and are frequently multiple. Though angiomyolipomas are uncommon in clinical practice nodules of smooth muscle and fat are found in the kidneys of 11 % of patients at post mortem. They are seen as well defined echogenic renal masses though uncommonly they have a low fat content in which case their echogenicity is reduced.

4.37.4 Renal papillary necrosis

Papillary necrosis is uncommon in adults and rare in children when there is usually clear evidence of an underlying cause such as chemotherapy. The renal papilla is very susceptible to ischaemic damage as blood in this area has a low oxygen tension. In adults papillary necrosis may be associated with infection, urinary obstruction, sickle cell disease, diabetes, analgesic abuse and other nephrotoxic drugs. In early cases the kidney appears normal sonographically. Advanced cases show juxta-calyceal cavities which may mimic hydronephrosis. A sloughed papilla may obstruct the ureter and cause hydronephrosis or give rise to a mass within the collecting system. Sloughed papillae may calcify and mimic stones.

4.38 PERI-RENAL FLUID COLLECTIONS

Abscess

Loculated ascites

Urinoma, anechoic fluid collection usually
    without septae or debris unless complicated
    by infection or haemorrhage. Most cases
    are secondary to obstruction, calculi,
    trauma, surgery or radiological intervention

Haematoma, may appear solid or fluid
    depending upon the stage of formation or
    liquefaction

Lymphocoeles. These are rare unless
    associated with renal transplantation

Seromas. Rare fluid collections, usually
    secondary to renal transplantation

Pseudocysts. Pancreatic or CSF pseudocysts
    may track into the perinephric spaces

Malignant infiltration. Infiltration with uniform
    malignant tissue may appear remarkably
    hypoechoic and be mistaken for a fluid
    collection. Lymphoma may completely
    encircle a kidney giving rise to a
    hypoechoic mantle

4.38.1 The ureters

The ureters lie on the anterior surface of psoas near
its medial edge. In the pelvis they cross anterior to the
common iliac vessels in front of the sacro-iliac joints.
They turn forwards at the level of the ischial spines
and in the female the ureter passes close to the lateral
fornix of vagina. The normal ureter is of small calibre
and is not usually visualized. When dilated the ureter
may be identified as a tubular fluid filled structure

continuous with the renal pelvis or lying behind the bladder. A dilated ureter may indent a partially filled bladder and may mimic a ureterocoele.

4.38.2 Megaureter in childhood

A Classification

Primary – non obstructive, non refluxing
Secondary – due to reflux, obstruction or obstruction masked by reflux

The patient usually presents with a urinary tract infection. The upper ureter is dilated though dilatation of the renal collecting system and lower ureter is variable. The underlying abnormality is lack of transmission of peristalsis in a short segment of ureter which may be narrowed. This may be due to a muscle anomaly, collagenous infiltration or an aganglionic segment of ureter analogous to Hirschsprungs disease of bowel.

4.38.3 Prune belly syndrome (Eagle Barrett syndrome)

The syndrome comprises deficiency of the abdominal musculature, cryptorchidism and urinary tract abnormality. The eventual prognosis depends upon the degree of underlying renal dysplasia and malformation. There is an intrinsic ureteric defect which gives rise to elongated tortuous ureters with upper tract dilatation. Ureteric dilatation is often massive and far greater than calyceal dilatation. Mild cases show only slight ureteric dilatation. Severe cases show fluid-filled flank masses representing dysplastic kidneys with ureteric dilatation.

4.38.4 Retroperitoneal fibrosis

Retroperitoneal fibrosis fixes the ureters and prevents
peristalsis leading to functional obstruction though the
ureteric lumen is not obliterated and a retrograde
catheter can be introduced via the bladder. Fibrosis
may be secondary to retroperitoneal haemorrhage,
tumour, inflammation or drug toxicity. The degree of
renal failure is usually far greater than suggested by
the degree of upper tract dilatation which may be
slight. A soft tissue mass may be present around the
great vessels. Unlike para-aortic lymphadenopathy the
mass does not usually distort the great vessels.

4.38.5 The urinary bladder

The urinary bladder is extraperitoneal and lies in the
pelvis though it is primarily an abdominal organ till six
years of age. The ureters pass obliquely through the
bladder wall the intramural course being 6–16 mm
long. The bladder wall thickness is usually between 3
and 6 mm when the bladder is distended.

A *Bladder wall*

   Transitional epithelium
   Submucous layer
   Muscle (detrusor)
   Subserous
   Serous/peritoneal

Sonographically the bladder is seen as an anechoic
sac of fluid in the anterior pelvis. Its shape, size and
wall thickness are very variable depending upon the
degree of distension.

4.38.6   Ureterocoele

A ureterocoele is a dilatation of the distal ureter which has herniated through the bladder wall into the bladder lumen. This usually occurs secondary to a distal ureteric stenosis which causes obstruction and dilatation of the distal ureter.

> Orthoptic (simple) ureterocoele: sited at the normal vesico-ureteric junction.
>
> Ectopic ureterocoele: these occur at sites of ectopic insertion of the ureter into the bladder, urethra, vagina, perineum etc. They usually arise at the ectopic insertion of the upper moiety ureter of a duplex kidney though a ureter from a non-duplex kidney can have an ectopic insertion. Ureterocoeles may be small or may be large enough to fill the entire bladder. They are dynamic structures which change shape depending upon the rate of urine production and degree of bladder distension.

A   Sonographic appearances

A ureterocoele is seen as an anechoic cyst-like fluid filled structure with a thin echogenic wall bulging into the bladder. Continuation with the dilated ureter is frequently evident.

4.38.7   Bladder diverticula

Bladder diverticula occur as protrusions of the bladder mucosa between the bundles of detrusor muscle. They are very variable in size and as they have no muscle in their walls they may increase in size during micturition. Congenital diverticula are uncommon and usually occur in boys. They occur more frequently secondary to bladder outflow obstruction or neurogenic bladder.

A *Sonographic appearances*

Diverticula are difficult to see when small but larger diverticula are seen as anechoic, fluid-filled structures around the bladder. Occasionally they may contain debris, clot, stones or tumour. They may be mistaken for ovarian cysts, bladder duplication, loculated ascites or a urachal remnant. Para-ureteric diverticula may distort the vesico-ureteric junction and cause reflux.

4.38.8 Cystitis

There are many causes of inflammation of the bladder wall including infection, radiation, drugs e.g. cyclophosphamide and trauma e.g. indwelling catheter or surgery. The bladder appears sonographically normal in the majority of cases but may show striking thickening of its wall due to oedema. (The bladder mucosa is normally less than 2 mm thick when measured at full distension.)

4.39 INTRALUMINAL BLADDER MASSES

(Including bladder wall lesions bulging into
   the lumen)

Bladder carcinoma
Benign prostatic hyperplasia
Prostatic malignancy
Clot
Calculi
Catheter
Foreign body
Bladder trabeculation
Rhabdomyosarcoma (usually children)
Localized haemorrhage or bladder wall
   oedema
Oedema at vesico-ureteric junction due to
   stone
Ureterocoele
Extension of adjacent malignancy
Abscess spreading to bladder wall
Endometriosis
Polyp
Fungus ball
Granuloma e.g. tuberculosis, schistosomiasis
Benign bladder wall tumour e.g.
>   Neurofibroma
>   Leiomyoma
>   Haemangioma
>   Phaeochromocytoma

Metastasis e.g.
>   Melanoma
>   Carcinoma of stomach
>   Breast carcinoma
>   Bronchial carcinoma

Leukoplakia

Cystitis cystica
Malakoplakia
Prolapsing urethral polyp

4.39.1 Bladder calculi

Bladder calculi are usually secondary to chronic incomplete bladder emptying and urine stasis. Calculi are seen as echogenic masses within the bladder lumen which are usually mobile and cause distal acoustic shadowing. Similar appearances occur with blood clot, foreign bodies and tumour encrusted with calcium salts.

Bladder calculi may be mimicked by subureteric teflon injection which gives rise to echogenic mounds which may shadow.

4.39.2 Bladder wall haematoma

Bladder wall haematomas are not uncommon if the bladder is examined sonographically immediately after instrumentation. Lesions may appear solid or cystic depending upon the nature of the blood. Focal oedema may also give rise to focal masses. Any such anomalies found after endoscopy should be followed up to ensure resolution.

4.39.3 Bladder tumours

Tumours of the bladder wall are seen as echogenic masses protruding into the bladder lumen from the wall. Transurethral scanning is the most accurate sonographic means of staging bladder tumours but is not usually practical. Superficial non-invasive tumours have a well defined base without bladder wall deformity or fixation. Tumour spreading into the bladder wall is seen as a hypoechoic area within the wall causing loss of continuity of normal wall echoes. More extensive tumour spread is seen as hypoechoic tumour extending into perivesical fat.

4.39.4 Neuropathic bladder

The bladder should be routinely scanned before and after micturition. Loss of normal neurological control of bladder function may affect bladder volume and appearance. Posterior nerve root lesions result in a large atonic bladder. Spinal cord lesions usually give rise to a spastic bladder which is trabeculated and may have multiple diverticula. In longstanding cases the bladder volume may be markedly reduced.

4.39.5 Bladder injury

The bladder is much more prone to injury in a child than in an adult owing to its abdominal position. It may be injured by blunt abdominal trauma, penetrating injury or pelvic fractures. The latter may also cause urethral injury.

    80 % of ruptures are extraperitoneal
    20 % of ruptures are intraperitoneal (higher in
        children)

Sonography may show fluid around the bladder or in the peritoneum.

4.40 PERIVESICAL FLUID

Pelvic ascites
Haematoma
Abscess/pus
Urinoma
Lymphocoele
Fluid in the pelvis post ovulation
Contrast post hysterosalpingography

4.40.1 The ureteral jet phenomenon

Urine enters the bladder intermittently as a jet propelled by a wave of peristalsis. If the urine entering the bladder differs in specific gravity compared to the urine already present then it may be visualized transiently as it enters the bladder as an echogenic stream which rapidly disperses and is lost in the urine already present. This phenomenon is seen most frequently when patients are given large volumes of fluid to drink prior to an ultrasound examination in order to fill the bladder. The average jet travels 3–5 cm and is seen 2–4 times a minute. The jet is usually at 45° to the posterior bladder wall but in 7 % of patients is at 90° to the posterior wall. Visualization of the jet allows localization of the vesico-ureteric junction and confirms that that kidney is producing urine.

4.40.2 The urachus

The urachus is a remnant of the allantois which connects the bladder to the umbilicus *in utero*. It may remain patent and give rise to cysts, sinuses or fistulae adjacent to the bladder apex though these are not usually visible sonographically. When a urachal cyst is seen it may appear solid or cystic and usually lies directly above the fundus of the bladder, often bulging into it.

4.40.3 Pelvic lipomatosis

Marked increase in the deposition of fat in the pelvis usually affects obese middle aged men. This results in bladder compression increasing its cranio-caudal length and narrowing it from side to side. The fat is seen as echogenic material filling the pelvis around the bladder. The majority of other diseases which result in bladder compression give rise to hypoechoic masses e.g.

Venous collaterals in IVC thrombosis
Bilateral iliac artery aneurysms
Lymphadenopathy
Pelvic tumours
Haematoma
Lymphocoele

The kidneys and ureters should be examined as aggressive fat deposition may cause upper tract obstruction.

4.40.4 The urethra

The urethra is not usually seen during bladder sonography though urethral diverticula have been diagnosed sonographically. Bladder outflow obstruction by urethral valves causes distension of the posterior urethra which may then be visualized. This is the commonest form of lower urinary tract obstruction in boys, it is very rare in girls.

A Classification of urethral valves

Type 1 – Exaggeration of plicae colliculi which extend from the verumontanum and attach to the anterolateral walls of the urethra

    Type 2 – Folds arising from the verumontanum
       which pass proximally to the bladder base. (May
       not be a true cause of obstruction)

    Type 3 – Diaphragm with a small central perforation.
       Situated proximal or distal to the verumontanum
       but not actually attached to it

The posterior urethra is dilated and visible in only
50 % of cases of posterior urethral valves if the bladder
is scanned at rest. Dilatation is more obvious if scanning
is undertaken during micturition. Other evidence of
bladder outflow obstruction includes bladder wall thickening and upper tract dilatation due to reflux or
retrograde transmission of increased bladder pressures.

4.41 THE ADRENAL GLANDS

The adrenal glands each weigh approximately 5 g and
measure $4 \times 2 \times 0.4$ cm in size. The right gland is
triangular or pyramidal in shape and lies in front of
the right crus of diaphragm behind the IVC and bare
area of liver at the upper pole of the right kidney. The
right crus of diaphragm may be mistaken for the adrenal
gland surrounded by perirenal fat. The left adrenal
gland is prerenal in position extending from the upper
pole of the left kidney almost down to the left renal
hilum. It lies in front of the left crus of diaphragm
behind the splenic vessels and pancreas and is crescentic
or semilunar in shape.

    Though the adrenal glands may be seen as slightly
echogenic bands, it is the fat around the adrenal which
is more frequently visualized. The adrenals appear
hypoechoic relative to the surrounding fat but they are
frequently only visualized when enlarged or calcified.
They may appear normal despite clinically proven

disease e.g. sonographic changes are only present in 50 % of proven cases of bilateral adrenal hyperplasia.

4.41.1 Adrenal masses

Small adrenal masses can frequently be visualized as they tend to be hypoechoic and are outlined by adjacent fat. Small masses lie antero-medial to the kidney whilst larger masses lie more anteriorly and may appear hepatic or renal in origin. Adrenal calcification is not uncommon and gives rise to echogenic foci within the gland. Bowel loops may be mistaken for adrenal masses but are inconstant when the patient's position is changed, particularly if the patient is scanned erect.

A *Adrenal tumours*

Lipoma, fibroma, cysts, angiomyolipoma – these are usually benign non-functioning tumours arising from connective tissue

Adenoma, carcinoma, gland hyperplasia – arise from the adrenal cortex

Phaeochromocytoma and neurogenic tumours – arise from the adrenal medulla

Metastases – particularly from breast, lung, ovary, melanoma, gastrointestinal and urinary tracts.

Tumour activity is not usually related to tumour size, e.g. small Conn's adenomas may be very active despite being too small to visualize sonographically. Benign tumours usually have a solid appearance with a well defined margin. Adrenal hyperplasia is difficult to identify and is easily mistaken for an adenoma if hyperplasia is nodular. Metastases are the commonest malignant adrenal lesions, they are usually hypoechoic but may be echogenic and are frequently bilateral.

Haemorrhage and necrosis give rise to a heterogenous appearance.

4.41.2 Neuroblastoma

Neuroblastoma is relatively common in children and is the commonest cause of a solid abdominal mass in a young child. Thirty per cent occur in the first year of life, frequency then decreases exponentially with age. Neuroblastoma is a malignant tumour derived from sympathetic neuroblast tissue, 70 % arise within the abdomen though only 37 % arise primarily within the adrenal glands. Neuroblastoma is a solid tumour which is often large at presentation. They have a more heterogenous echopattern than Wilms tumour and calcific foci are frequently seen both in the primary tumour and metastases. The tumour may metastasize to the liver directly or via the blood stream. Cases of neuroblastoma frequently present with evidence of metastases before the primary tumour is evident. In these cases ultrasonography is invaluable at demonstrating adrenal pathology.

A Differential diagnosis

Tuberculoma may give identical appearances but usually affects an older age group and is quite rare in the United Kingdom. Wilms tumour is the main differential diagnosis and in cases of suspected neuroblastoma the kidney usually appears normal though it may be displaced.

4.41.3 Adrenal carcinoma

Adrenal carcinoma is usually large at diagnosis as symptoms occur late even when the tumour is functional. (Carcinomas demonstrate less endocrine function than adenomas relative to their size.) They occur less frequently than adrenal metastases. A heterogenous mass is the commonest appearance though haemorrhage and necrosis may give rise to cystic areas with thick irregular walls. The mass is generally hypoechoic compared to normal adrenal tissue. The renal vein, IVC and retroperitoneum should be inspected for evidence of tumour spread. The liver is also a frequent site of metastases.

4.41.4 Adrenal cysts

Adrenal cysts are found in 6 % of patients at post mortem but are usually too small to be visualized sonographically. The majority are asymptomatic and are thus of little clinical relevance. They occur more frequently in women than in men.

A *Aetiology*

Lymphangioma. (Endothelial) May be multilocular and can be huge
Epithelial cysts
Embryonic cystic adenomas
Pseudocysts. Due to liquefaction of haematoma. They occur most frequently in the neonate
Necrotic tumour
Infection, e.g. hydatid cyst

4.41.5 Phaeochromocytoma

These are neurogenic tumours which arise from the adrenal medulla or sympathetic chain. They are usually benign but 10 % are malignant, 10 % are multiple and

10 % arise outside the adrenal. (Ninety per cent of these are within the abdomen.) Sonographic appearances are of a solid mass of variable size with a hypoechoic or heterogenous echopattern.

4.41.6   Adrenal haemorrhage

The majority of cases occur in the neonate, usually between the second and seventh days of life. The haematoma may have a solid or cystic appearance depending upon the stage of haematoma formation or liquefaction. Longstanding cases may calcify giving a densely echogenic appearance with shadowing. In neonates calcification may be present as early as 10 days after haemorrhage. Adrenal haemorrhage may occur *in utero* and bilateral adrenal calcification may be present at birth.

4.41.7   Angiomyolipoma

Angiomyolipoma of the adrenal gland is seen as an echogenic mass, its appearance being identical to angiomyolipoma of the kidney.

4.41.8   Myelolipoma

Myelolipoma is a rare tumour which contains fat and bone marrow elements. Sonographically it is seen as an echogenic mass which is hypovascular on angiography. Computerized tomography may suggest the diagnosis as the fat content may be demonstrated.

4.42 ANECHOIC SUPRARENAL MASSES

Adrenal haemorrhage
Cyst (adrenal, renal, hepatic, splenic, mesenteric)
Hydronephrosis of upper moiety of a duplex kidney
Abscess
Necrotic tumour (adrenal or renal)
Cystic neuroblastoma
Hydatid cyst

4.43 BILATERAL ADRENAL MASSES

Metastases (most frequent)
Adrenal hyperplasia
Bilateral phaeochromocytoma
Adrenal cysts
Adrenal haematomas

FURTHER READING

Abu-Yousef M M *et al*. Bladder tumours studied by cystosonography. *Radiology* (1984) **153**: 223–226.

Abu-Yousef M M *et al*. Urinary bladder tumours studied by cystosonography. Part 2 staging. *Radiology* (1984) **153**: 227–231.

Amis E S & Hartman D S. Renal ultrasonography. *Rad. Clin. North Am*. (1984) **22**(2): 315–332.

Amis E S Jr *et al*. Ultrasonic inaccuracies in diagnosing renal obstruction. *Urology* (1982) **19**: 101–105.

Bartum R J *et al*. The ultrasonic determination of renal transplant volume. *J. Clin. Ult*. (1974) **2**(4): 281–285.

Bartum R J *et al*. Evaluation of renal transplant with ultrasound. *Radiology* (1976) **118**: 405–410.

Birnholz J C *et al*. Submucosal oedema of the collecting system. A new ultrasonic sign of severe renal allograft rejection. *Radiology* (1985) **154**: 190.

Bisset R A L & Khan A N. Detection of active bleeding from a transitional cell carcinoma of the bladder by ultrasonography. *J. Clin. Ult.* (1987) **15**: 269–272.

Blake N S & O'Connell E. Endoscopic correction of vesico-ureteric reflux by sub-ureteric Teflon injection. Follow up ultrasonography and voiding cystography. *Brit. J. Rad.* (1989) **62**: 443–446.

Blase C E *et al*. Sonographic standards for normal infant kidney length. *Am. J. Roent.* (1985) **145**: 1289–1291.

Bortstein Y *et al*. Leiomyoma of the bladder: sonographic and urographic findings. *J. Ult. Med.* (1986) **5**: 407–408.

Carter K M *et al*. Renal ultrasonography in Beckwith Wiedermann syndrome. *Paed. Rad.* (1981) **11**: 46–48.

Chippindale A J *et al*. Case report: 2 patients with symptomatic renal metastases. *Clin. Rad.* (1989) **40**: 95–97.

Cochlin D *et al*. Ultrasound changes in the transplanted kidney. *Clin. Rad.* (1988) **39**: 373–376.

Cochran S T *et al*. Nephromegaly in hyperalimentation. *Radiology* (1979) **130**: 603–606.

Conrad M R *et al*. New observations in renal transplant using ultrasound. *Am. J. Roent.* (1978) **131**: 851–855.

Cronan J J *et al*. Cystosonography in the detection of bladder tumours: a prospective and retrospective study. *J. Ult. Med.* (1982) **145**: 611–616.

Diamont M J *et al*. Hydronephrosis in childhood: reliability of ultrasound screening. *Paed. Rad.* (1984) **14**: 31–36.

Friedland G W *et al.* (eds) *Uroradiology, an Integrated Approach* Churchill Livingstone (1983).

Goldberg B B. *Abdominal Ultrasonography*, 2nd ed, p. 326. John Wiley & Sons (1984).

Gordillo R *et al.* Circumscribed renal mass in a dysplastic kidney: pseudotumour vs tumour. *J. Ult. Med.* (1987) **6**: 613–617.

Hamper U M *et al.* Renal involvement in AIDS sonographic – pathologic correlation. *Am. J. Roent.* (1988) **150**: 1321–1325.

Han B K & Babcock D S. Sonographic measurements and appearance of normal kidneys in children. *Am. J. Roent.* (1985) **145**: 611–616.

Hartman D S *et al.* Renal lymphoma: radiologic – pathologic correlation of 21 cases. *Radiology* (1982) **144**: 759–766.

Hendry G M A. Cystic neuroblastoma of the adrenal gland, a potential source of error in ultrasonic diagnosis. *Paed. Rad.* (1982) **12**: 204–206.

Khan A N *et al.* Primary renal liposarcoma mimicking angiomyolipoma on ultrasonography and conventional radiology. *J. Clin. Ult.* (1985) **13**: 58–59.

Lafortune M *et al.* Sonography of the hypertrophied column of Bertin. *Am. J. Roent.* (1986) **146**: 53–56.

Lang E K. (ed.) *Current Concepts of Uroradiology (International Perspectives in Urology vol 9)* Williams and Wilkins (1984).

Leopold G R. Renal transplant size measured by reflected ultrasound. *Radiology* (1970) **95**: 687–689.

McCullough D L & Leopold G R. Diagnosis of retroperitoneal fluid collections by ultrasonography: a series of surgically proved cases. *J. Urol.* (1976) **115**: 656–659.

Nardi P M *et al.* Renal manifestations of Kawasaki's disease. *Paed. Rad.* (1985) **15**: 116–118.

Pickering S P *et al*. Renal lymphangioma: a cause of neonatal nephromegaly. *Paed. Rad.* (1984) **14**: 445–448.

Rao T K S *et al*. Associated focal and segmental glomerulosclerosis in the acquired immunodeficiency syndrome. *N. Eng. J. Med.* (1974) **290**: 19–23.

Rosenbaum D M *et al*. Sonographic assessment of renal length in normal children. *Am. J. Roent.* (1984) **142**: 467–469.

Rosenfield A T *et al*. Ultrasound in experimental and clinical renal vein thrombosis. *Radiology* (1980) **137**: 735–741.

Rosenfield A T *et al*. Clinical applications of ultrasound tissue characterisation. *Rad. Clin. North Am.* (1980) **18**(1): 31–58.

Sanders R C. *Atlas of ultrasonographic artefacts and variants.* Yearbook publications (1986).

Saxton H. Myths and misconceptions in uroradiology. *Clin. Rad.* (1988) **39**: 361–362.

Silverman P M *et al*. Adrenal sonography in renal agenesis and dysplasia. *Am. J. Roent.* (1980) **134**: 600–602.

Suzuki T *et al*. Sonography of cyclophosphamide cystitis: a report of 2 cases. *J. Clin. Ult.* (1988) **16**: 183–187.

Weill F S *et al*. Pseudotumours in normal kidney. *Renal Sonography* 2nd ed. Springer-Verlag (1987).

Worthington J L *et al*. Sonographically detectable cysts in polycystic kidney disease in newborn and young infants. *Paed. Rad.* (1988) **18**: 287–293.

Yeh H C *et al*. Ultrasonography of renal sinus lipomatosis. *Radiology* (1977) **124**: 799–801.

Chapter 5

Male Genital Tract

5.1 THE MALE GENITAL TRACT

The adult testis is an ovoid structure measuring 4–5 cm × 3 cm × 2.5 cm. It has a smooth homogenous parenchyma returning mid-amplitude echoes though small echogenic foci may also be seen. The epididymis lies on the posterolateral aspect of the testis. It has a coarser echopattern than the testis but is of similar echogenicity. It may be differentiated from the testis by two parallel echogenic lines. The head of the epididymis lies superiorly and is slightly more echogenic than the testis. A small volume of fluid is frequently seen around the testis lying between the parietal and visceral layers of the tunica vaginalis.

5.1.1 Hydrocoele

A hydrocoele is the commonest cause of scrotal swelling. It is usually painless and without treatment may become very large. The majority of hydrocoeles are idiopathic but they may be secondary to any scrotal pathology such as testicular tumour, trauma, torsion or inflammation. Sonographically the hydrocoele is seen as an anechoic fluid collection around the testicle except posteriorly at the site of attachment of the epididymis. The presence of fluid makes assessment of testicular echogenicity unreliable and the testicle may appear abnormally echogenic relative to the fluid. Longstanding cases may be associated with thickening of the tunica vaginalis and infection or haemorrhage may give rise to internal septae or debris. Sonographic appearances may be identical to para-testicular abscess or haematocoele and these must be differentiated on clinical grounds or by aspiration. Loculated hydrocoeles may also occur along the course of the processus vaginalis. If the processus vaginalis fails to close the hydrocoele may be seen to extend into the pelvis.

5.1.2 Varicocoele

A varicocoele is a collection of tortuous dilated veins arising from the pampiniform venous plexus. Normal spermatic cord veins measure from 0.5–1.5 mm in diameter with a main draining vein up to 2 mm in diameter. The veins forming a varicocoele are usually uniform in size measuring up to 5 mm in diameter. Vessel size increases if the patient is scanned when standing or performing a Valsalva manoeuvre. Over 95 % of cases occur on the left, the occurrence of a varicocoele on the right should raise the possibility of underlying abdominal pathology. The right testicular vein drains to the I.V.C. but the left vein drains to the left renal vein thus a left-sided varicocoele can be secondary to renal carcinoma.

5.1.3 Spermatocoele

Spermatocoeles are usually solitary and arise in the region of the head of epididymis. They are lobulated sonolucent collections 2–3 cm in diameter.

5.1.4 Epididymal cyst

An epididymal cyst also has the appearance of a sonolucent fluid collection but these cysts tend to occur in the body of the epididymis.

5.1.5 Hernia

Herniation of bowel through the inguinal canal is the commonest cause of inguinal swelling. Bowel loops may reach the scrotum and may be recognized sonographically when fluid filled as they will show peristalsis on prolonged examination. When filled with air they will appear echogenic with shadowing.

5.1.6 The undescended testicle

The testes arise on the posterior abdominal wall and descend into the scrotum late in foetal life. There is maldescent of the testes in 0.23–0.8 % of males and it is bilateral in 10–25 % of cases. At birth 4 % of testes have failed to reach the scrotum but the incidence falls to 0.8 % by six weeks of age. Lack of normal descent increases the risk of trauma, torsion and tumour and is also associated with decreased fertility. Seventy per cent of undescended testicles lie in the inguinal canal and these may be seen as hypoechoic structures relative to adjacent soft tissues. They are smaller than a normal gonad due to testicular atrophy. Testicles lying on the lateral pelvic wall can sometimes be identified but are frequently obscured by bowel gas.

5.1.7 Testicular trauma

Clinical examination is an unreliable means of assessing testicular integrity particularly if the testicle is surrounded by haematoma. Ultrasonography allows visualization of the testicle despite the presence of haematoma though rupture may still be difficult to identify unless the testicle is fragmented or extrusion of testicular material is shown. Haemorrhage within the testicle may be seen as anechoic blood or echogenic clot. Infarction may be identical. An established haematoma may give a bizarre complex mass appearance. Without a history of trauma the appearances are similar to those of infarction, abscess and tumour and haemorrhage is more likely to occur if the testicle is already diseased.

5.1.8 Torsion of the testis

Testicular torsion usually presents with acute pain and swelling but may present as painless scrotal swelling particularly in young children. Surgery must be performed within 6 h of the onset of symptoms if function is to be preserved. In the early stages the testicle appears normal. It then becomes swollen and may appear of increased or decreased echogenicity. Six hours after the onset of symptoms the testis is normally hypoechoic and a normal scan at this time makes torsion unlikely. Doppler studies may show decreased or absent flow in the testicular artery. The testis may also appear rather high in the scrotum and may be noted to have a rather horizontal axis.

If the testicular torsion is not treated surgically in the acute phase the hypoechoic testicle becomes enlarged and a hydrocoele may develop. The testicle then atrophies making the epididymis appear relatively large and echogenic in comparison. The main differential diagnosis of testicular torsion in clinical practice is that of epididymo-orchitis, in the acute stage sonography may not be able to differentiate these two conditions and isotope scanning may be more valuable if available.

5.1.9 Epididymitis/orchitis

Epididymo-orchitis is the commonest intra-scrotal inflammation. Sonographic appearances are variable depending upon the stage and severity of the disease. The epididymis is usually enlarged and hypoechoic but it may be intensely echogenic. In uncomplicated cases of epididymitis the testicle is usually not involved though there may be hypoechoic foci in the testicular parenchyma adjacent to the epididymis. Orchitis gives rise to hypoechoic foci and in severe cases results in an enlarged hypoechoic testicle with secondary hydrocoele formation. In chronic epididymitis the epididymis becomes echogenic and in tuberculous epididymitis it may be stony hard and calcified.

5.1.10 Testicular tumours

Testicular tumours occur most frequently in the 20–40 year age group. Their incidence is increased 5–100 times in undescended testicles and orchidopexy after the age of six years does not appear to reduce this risk. Fifteen per cent of testicular tumours present with a hydrocoele whilst others present with a testicular mass or distant metastases. Tumours are usually classified by germ cell (e.g. seminoma and teratoma) and non-germ cell origin. Seminoma is the commonest testicular tumour in adults whilst teratoma is the commonest in

children. Over the age of 50 years 50 % of testicular
neoplasms are lymphomas. Metastases also occur particularly from lung, leukaemia, prostate, melanoma
and neuroblastoma. Over 90 % of testicular neoplasms
are completely or predominantly hypoechoic. Infarction and inflammation may also give rise to focal
hypoechoic areas and thus a hypoechoic focus does
not necessarily indicate malignancy. High frequency
sonography is a very accurate means of demonstrating
testicular parenchyma and a normal scan is almost
100 % accurate at excluding testicular malignancy.

5.2   ECHOPOOR TESTICULAR LESIONS

Tumour
Orchitis
Torsion
Abscess
Haemorrhage
Focal infarction
Granuloma

A   *Seminoma*
Accounts for 50 % of primary neoplasms. Usually gives
rise to a well defined hypoechoic mass.

B   *Teratoma*
Accounts for less than 10 % of primary neoplasms. It
may appear primarily solid, cystic or complex. The
presence of cartilage and bony elements may give rise
to echogenic areas with shadowing.

C   *Embryonal cell carcinoma*
Commonest appearance is of a hypoechoic mass with
irregular borders which may show echogenic foci due
to areas of calcification.

D Choriocarcinoma

This rare tumour is rapidly fatal. It usually gives rise to a complex mass with cystic areas due to haemorrhage and necrosis and may also have echogenic foci due to calcification.

E Lymphoma

Gives rise to a homogenous hypoechoic mass similar to seminoma. Leukaemic deposits also give a similar appearance.

Synchronous or metachronous tumours occur in 2 % of patients and thus both testicles should always be examined. Intratesticular lesions should be considered malignant till proven otherwise but homogenous echogenic lesions are usually benign e.g. lipoma, adenomatoid tumour, fibrous scar, old infarct.

5.3 TOTALLY CYSTIC SCROTAL MASS

Hydrocoele
Spermatocoele
Epididymal cyst
Haematoma
Varicocoele (usually shows multiple anechoic
  channels)
Abscess
Fluid filled bowel loop

5.4 SOLID SCROTAL MASS

Testicular mass e.g. tumour, inflamed testicle
Inflamed epididymis
Bowel loop
Scrotal wall tumour

5.4.1 The prostate

Though the prostate may be visualized on abdominal
scanning it is seen most clearly on rectal scanning. It
has a heterogenous slightly echogenic central zone
surrounded by a more homogenous slightly hypoechoic
peripheral zone. The lower echogenicity of the peripheral zone is due to its higher muscle content. This zone
comprises the posterior, apical and lateral lobes and is
the site of origin of 70 % of prostatic carcinomas. The
seminal vesicles can often be visualized lying behind
and slightly above the prostate. They are hypoechoic
relative to adjacent prostatic parenchyma.

A Benign prostatic hyperplasia

The size of the prostate increases in middle-aged and
elderly males. As it enlarges the prostate becomes

asymmetrical and bulges upwards into the bladder. Hypertrophy it usually most prominent in the central zone. The enlarged gland may have a homogenous echopattern but may appear heterogenous particularly if previously affected by prostatitis or if complicated by areas of infarction, ductal dilatation or stone formation.

5.4.2 Prostatic tumours

At post mortem 12–46 % of men over 50 years of age have foci of prostatic carcinoma on gland histology. The incidence rises further to reach 90 % by the age of 90 years. The clinical incidence of prostatic carcinoma is far lower and the natural history of the disease is not fully understood at present. Over 70 % of primary prostatic malignancies arise in the peripheral zone of the gland causing loss of normal gland symmetry and echotexture. Prostatic carcinoma does not have a specific sonographic appearance though most tumours are hypoechoic. Calcification occurs giving rise to echogenic foci.

A *General appearances of prostatic carcinoma*

54 % of lesions are echolucent
22 % of lesions are echopoor
24 % of lesions are isoechoic.

Later series state that over 90 % of prostatic carcinomas are hypoechoic and nearly 100 % of extensive tumours are hypoechoic.

Transrectal sonography with simultaneous prostatic biopsy via a perineal approach allows accurate tissue diagnosis of prostatic lesions. Ultrasonography is also a valuable means of disease staging as extension of carcinoma through the gland capsule may be readily demonstrated with loss of capsular continuity and gland outline. Most predominantly hypoechoic lesions prove to be malignant whilst predominantly hyperechoic areas are rarely malignant. Sonography may follow up these tumours, therapy usually results in an increase in parenchyma echogenicity.

5.4.3 Prostatitis

Prostatic inflammation gives rise to tender enlargement of the gland which has a rather soft consistency on palpation. In acute prostatitis the gland may be of normal size but it is often enlarged and deformed. The capsular margin becomes ill-defined and the enlarged gland shows hypoechoic areas. The presence of calculi within the gland parenchyma gives rise to echogenic foci. With treatment the gland size and contour return to normal but the abnormal echotexture may persist. In chronic prostatitis the gland shows a persistently abnormal echopattern which may be heterogenously echogenic with evidence of calculi which usually lie posterior to the urethra and in the gland periphery. (Calculi tend to occur around the urethra in urethritis.)

FURTHER READING

Arger P H *et al*. Prospective analysis of the value of scrotal ultrasound. *Radiology* (1981) **141**: 763–766.

Carroll B A & Gross D M. High frequency scrotal sonography. *Am. J. Roent.* (1983) **140**: 511–512.

Clements R *et al*. How accurate is the index finger. A comparison of digital and ultrasound examination of the prostatic nodule. *Clin. Rad.* (1988) **39**: 87–89.

Coleman B G. *Genitourinary Ultrasound: A Text/Atlas*. Igaku-Shoin (1988).

Cunningham J J. Sonographic findings in clinically unsuspected acute and chronic scrotal haematocoeles. *Am. J. Roent.* (1983) **140**: 749–752.

Griffiths G J *et al*. The ultrasound appearances of prostatic cancer with histological correlation. *Clin. Rad.* (1987) **38**: 219–227.

Griffiths G J *et al*. Ultrasonic appearances associated with prostatic inflammation: a preliminary study. *Clin. Rad.* (1984) **35**: 343–345.

Jeffrey R B *et al*. Sonography of testicular trauma. *Am. J. Roent.* (1983) **141**: 993–995.

Leopold G R *et al*. High resolution ultrasonography of scrotal pathology. *Radiology* (1979) **131**: 719–722.

Madrazo B L *et al*. Ultrasonographic demonstration of undescended testes. *Radiology* (1979) **133**: 181–183.

Schwerk W B *et al*. Testicular tumours: prospective analysis of real-time ultrasound patterns and abdominal staging. *Radiology* (1987) **164**: 369–374.

Wolverson M K *et al*. High resolution real-time sonography of scrotal varicocoele. *Am. J. Roent.* (1983) **141**: 775–779.

Chapter 6

Female Genital Tract

6.1 THE UTERUS

The foetus is subject to the influence of maternal hormones and thus at birth the neonatal uterus has a similar configuration to the post-pubertal uterus. The average neonatal uterine size is: length 3.4 cm, width 1.25 cm.

In the majority of cases endometrial echoes may be demonstrated. Over the next few weeks the uterus involutes to achieve the normal prepubertal configuration measuring: length 2–3.3 cm, width 0.5–1 cm.

At this stage the body and cervix of uterus are of similar length giving a body : cervix ratio of 1 : 1. After puberty the ratio increases to 2 : 1. The uterine size remains relatively stable till seven years of age and then increases in size and volume. At puberty it assumes the adult configuration with a pear shape and average dimensions of: length 5–8 cm, width 1.6–3 cm.

Uterine volume is approximately $\frac{1}{2} \times$ length $\times$ width $\times$ breadth. Uterine volume in a prepubertal girl is usually < 2 ml and often < 1 ml. It rapidly increases to around 25 ml at puberty. The body of uterus is anteflexed or angled slightly fowards in relation to the cervix. The whole uterus is usually anteverted forwards 90° in relation to the long axis of the vagina though it may be retroverted in up to 10 % of women. The retroverted uterus lies deep in the pelvis and is more difficult to evaluate sonographically than the anteverted uterus. During pregnancy the uterus increases in size up to 30 times by muscle fibre hypertrophy. After pregnancy it involutes but usually remains larger than before.

6.1.1 Uterine malformations

Congenital uterine malformations are found in 0.1–0.5 % of women and they may be associated with congenital anomalies of the urinary tract due to their similar embryological origins. These anomalies may be visualized sonographically and the diagnosis confirmed by hysterosalpingography. (Fig. 14.)

A Uterine hypoplasia
Hypoplasia of the uterus is not usually evident clinically until puberty. Causes include lack of oestrogens, chromosomal anomalies and *in-utero* exposure to diethylstilboestrol.

B Effects of diethylstilboestrol (DES) exposure *in utero*

Increased risk of clear cell carcinoma of the vagina (though this is still rare)
Genital anomalies including:
vaginal adenosis 35 %
vaginal fibrous ridges 22 %
abnormal vaginal mucosa 56 %
small T shaped uterus 14 %

6.1.2 Intra-uterine contraceptive devices

Intra-uterine contraceptive devices (IUCDs) are seen as echogenic structures which should lie within the

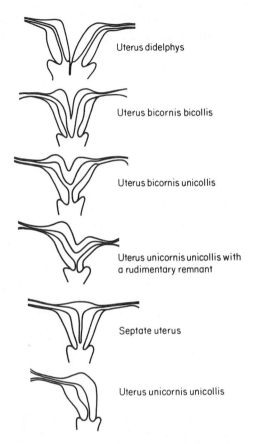

Uterus didelphys

Uterus bicornis bicollis

Uterus bicornis unicollis

Uterus unicornis unicollis with a rudimentary remnant

Septate uterus

Uterus unicornis unicollis

Fig. 14. Congenital uterine anomalies.

central uterine canal though they may protrude into or through the uterine wall. The central uterine canal is usually seen as a linear echogenic structure in the middle of the uterus running from the cervix to the fundus. IUCDs are also seen as linear echogenic structures (though curved IUCDs may be seen as a series of echogenic dots) usually within the central canal. They remain echogenic even at very low gain settings provided that care is taken to ensure that the IUCD is at the centre of the ultrasound beam. Entry and exit echoes from both walls of the IUCD may give rise to parallel line echoes and occasionally there may be distal acoustic shadowing.

A Features of IUCDs

High amplitude echoes in the uterine cavity
Echoes remain at low gain settings
Entrance and exit echoes giving a parallel line appearance are seen in 65 % of cases
± Distal acoustic shadowing
Configuration of echoes reflects the type of IUCD

B Differential diagnosis

Central cavity echoes – lost at low gain settings
Air in uterine canal e.g. post instrumentation
Other foreign body

6.1.3 Endometriosis

Endometriosis is the presence of endometrial tissue outside the endometrial lining of the uterus. Endometrial tissue is found within the myometrium in 10–50 % of menstruating females at post mortem. In only 10 % of cases is the ectopic endometrium capable of undergoing cyclical bleeding. At pelvic surgery 8–20 % of women have evidence of endometriosis. Endometriosis is thus a very common condition but the majority of deposits are small, are unlikely to cause symptoms and are not detectable sonographically.

A Sonographic appearances

Recurrent bleeding may give rise to cystic areas with variable internal echoes which may mimic solid masses

Irregular cystic spaces – chocolate cyst – thick walled discrete mass with irregular borders and low level internal echoes which may give a solid or complex appearance. These may occur distant to the uterus

Hypoechoic focal enlargement of the uterine wall

Irregular uterine shape

Thickening of posterior myometrium, may be mistaken for fibroids

Distortion of the endometrial cavity

6.2 ENDOMETRIOSIS – DIFFERENTIAL DIAGNOSIS

Uterine fibroids

Nabothian cysts – small fluid filled spaces in the myometrium near the cervix due to retention cysts of the cervical glands

Cystic and solid ovarian tumours

Tubo-ovarian abscess

Uterine tumours

Pelvic inflammatory disease

Ectopic pregnancy

Haemorrhagic cyst

6.3 ENDOMETRIAL FLUID COLLECTIONS

Prepubertal and adolescent:	Haematometra and congenital uterine anomalies
Adult:	Pregnancy and its complications
Post-menopausal:	Pelvic malignancy Endometrial polyps Chronic inflammation Cervical stenosis (benign or malignant)

6.3.1 Asherman's syndrome

Adhesions in the uterine canal or absence of the uterine canal due to damage during delivery/pregnancy/curettage. Sonography may show a normal shaped uterus with no cavity, haematosalpinx or haematometra.

6.3.2 Endometritis

Bacterial inflammation of the endometrium may occur post-partum, following abortion or due to the presence of intra-uterine contraceptive devices. The uterus may appear normal or may be enlarged with a wide echogenic canal which may contain fluid or air. (Air is not normally present within the uterine canal more than three days after instrumentation.) Fluid may also be present in the pelvis.

6.3.3 Uterine fibroids

Uterine fibroids or leiomyoma are localized proliferations of smooth muscle. These are often multiple causing lobular uterine enlargement. They may be complicated by haemorrhage and degeneration and may increase in size during pregnancy. Sonographically they are usually seen as masses in or arising from the myometrium. They are usually relatively homogenous and hypoechoic relative to normal myometrium. Haemorrhage and necrosis complicate the appearance giving rise to anechoic areas or a heterogenous appearance and calcification may give rise to echogenic foci with shadowing. Pedunculated fibroids protrude from the uterus and may give rise to adnexal masses indistinguishable from ovarian carcinoma. Pedunculated fibroids protruding internally from the myometrium may prolapse through the cervix to reach the vagina.

6.3.4 Uterine tumours

Uterine tumours are rare before puberty and at this age they are nearly all malignant. At this age rhabdomyosarcoma is the most frequent. This gives rise to a predominantly hypoechoic mass. The majority of uterine tumours occur in adults arising at the endocervix or within the endometrium of the body of uterus. Cervical cancer is usually diagnosed clinically without sonographic examination which may be normal but may show an enlarged distorted uterus with deformity of the cervix. Cervical stenosis may cause haematometra.

Endometrial cancer occurs most frequently in postmenopausal women. Sonography may be normal or may show an enlarged lobulated uterus with an abnormal echotexture and distorted canal.

6.4 THE VAGINA

Provided the urinary bladder is adequately filled the vagina is virtually always visible. The anterior and posterior walls are usually in apposition giving a slit-like appearance in transverse section. In longitudinal section the walls are seen as parallel hypoechoic bands separated by a central echogenic band representing the mucosa and lumen.

True absence of the vagina is rare, this clinical appearance is usually due to labial or vaginal adhesions. Congenital vaginal obstruction may occur due to the presence of a membrane just proximal to the hymen. Rarely a membrane may occur at the junction of the upper and middle thirds of the vagina at the point of fusion of the Mullerian duct and sinus derivatives. Vaginal obstruction by a membrane may cause haematocolpos in the newborn or haematometrocolpos in menstruating girls. Sonography may show the area of obstruction and dilatation of the proximal vagina and uterus.

6.4.1 Vaginal masses

A Cystic masses

Haematocolpos

Gartner duct cysts. These usually lie proximal to the vagina in the adnexa or along the antero-lateral aspect of the vaginal wall. They arise from Mesonephric duct remnants and are the commonest cystic vaginal lesions. They are usually incidental findings

Para-urethral cysts
Urethral diverticula
Inclusion cysts
Paramesonephric duct cysts
Cystocoeles
Ureterocoeles

B Solid masses

Foreign body e.g. tampon (appearance is variable, may be seen as a very echogenic mass with shadowing but when soaked in fluid the texture of the material may be discernable). The possibility of a foreign body should always be remembered in children who may give no history of insertion of the article which may have been present for some time.

Fibroids. Hypoechoic mass prolapsing through the cervix

Tumours. True vaginal tumours are rare in children and uncommon in adults. Clear cell carcinoma may be associated with DES exposure *in utero*. Primary and secondary tumours are usually seen as solid heterogenous masses

6.5 THE OVARIES

The ovaries develop on the posterior abdominal wall adjacent to the kidneys but descend into the pelvis as the kidneys ascend. They can thus lie high in the abdomen but usually lie along the superior margin of the broad ligament at birth. The ovaries measure 1.5 × 0.3 × 0.25 mm at birth and are usually not identified until two years of age. Over five years of age they can be identified in the majority of patients. Ovarian volume is relatively constant from birth to five years of age but over five years there is an age related increase in volume. Prepubertal ovarian volume is 0.3–0.9 cm^3.

At puberty the ovaries enlarge with volume increasing to 1.8–5.7 cm^3 and size ranging from 2.4–4.1 × 1.5–2.4 × 0.85–1.94 cm. As the ovaries enlarge at puberty they descend further into the pelvis. Under six years of age the ovary has a homogenous echotexture but over six years of age microcysts begin to form. (These may sometimes be seen in neonates due to the action of maternal hormones.) The adult ovary is an almond shaped organ which contains multiple small anechoic follicles in which the ova develop. During each menstrual cycle one follicle becomes dominant and enlarges. At ovulation the dominant follicle has an average size of around 2 cm. After release of the ovum the follicle regresses and rapidly shrinks. Immediately after follicle rupture a small amount of free fluid may be visible in the pelvis. Serial ultrasound scans charting follicular growth allow accurate prediction of ovulation in the majority of patients. Errors may occur with the development of corpus luteum cysts post-ovulation, reappearance of a follicle post-ovulation or haemorrhage into a follicle. Follicles associated with hormone-induced ovulation tend to be larger than normal. Excessive hormone therapy results in the formation of large ovarian cysts with bilateral ovarian enlargement. This may be associated with ascites, pleural effusions, electrolyte disturbances and blood volume changes.

6.5.1 Lack of visualization of the ovary

Normal ovary obscured by bowel. Bladder may be inadequately distended or over distended

Small ovaries e.g. Turmer's syndrome

Mullerian dysgenesis

Ectopic ovary e.g. ovary herniated into inguinal canal failure of normal descent, ovary in the lower abdomen

Small ovary post menopause

6.5.2 Ovarian masses

Small ovarian cysts are physiological and may be up to 3 cm in diameter just before ovulation. They have the appearance of simple cysts unless haemorrhage occurs in which case they may appear echogenic, mixed, septate, hypoechoic or anechoic. In cases of doubt the patient should be re-examined as physiological cysts show changing dimensions and usually resolve after ovulation. Cysts complicated by haemorrhage may be impossible to differentiate from other cystic or solid ovarian masses. Diagnosis is further complicated by the fact that 5–17 % of women with polycystic ovaries develop ovarian tumours.

6.6 DIFFERENTIAL DIAGNOSIS OF CYSTIC OVARIAN MASSES

Follicular cysts
Para ovarian cysts
Corpus luteum cysts
Theca lutein cysts
Ectopic pregnancy
Endometriosis
Haematoma
Adnexal torsion
Peritoneal and mesenteric cysts
Polycystic ovary syndrome
Cystic ovarian tumours
Tubo-ovarian abscess and pelvic inflammatory
  disease
Bowel loop
Loculated ascites
Appendix abscess
Dermoid
Degenerated fibroid

6.6.1 Ovarian cysts

A Follicular cysts

If a dominant follicle fails to ovulate it may remain active but immature. Less stimulated follicles may also fail to regress. Follicular cysts are usually small being around 1–1.5 cm in diameter but they are often multiple. Cysts are thin walled and occur in an otherwise normal ovary. If these cysts persist they may be associated with endometrial hyperplasia.

B Corpus luteum cyst

After fertilization of the ovum the follicle persists as a corpus luteum which produces hormones necessary to maintain the early pregnancy. Corpus luteum cysts are usually smooth walled anechoic or hypoechoic structures though they may give the appearance of a complex adnexal mass. They may rupture causing severe lower abdominal pain and serious intra-peritoneal haemorrhage in early pregnancy. This complication may mimic ectopic pregnancy.

C Theca lutein cysts

Theca lutein cysts are usually secondary to an underlying disorder such as hydatidiform mole, choriocarcinoma or hormonal therapy for anovulation. They are usually bilateral, thick walled, well-defined septate structures up to 10 cm in diameter.

D Haemorrhagic ovarian cyst

Benign and malignant ovarian cysts may be complicated by haemorrhage. The sonographic appearance is very variable depending upon the state of the blood within the cyst. Fresh blood is anechoic but rapidly becomes echogenic as it clots. The cyst may appear anechoic, solid, complex or septate and debris levels may be present.

E Polycystic ovary

Patients with polycystic ovaries may have amenorrhoea, infertility, obestity and hirsutism though not all these features are present in each case. The syndrome occurs due to a self-perpetuating hormonal disorder. Rarely there is an underlying pituitary abnormality. Thirty per cent of patients have normal-sized ovaries though serial examinations will show that the follicles fail to change size or configuration with time. Seventy per cent of patients have enlarged ovaries up to three times the normal size with three overall patterns:

Discrete cysts
Hypoechoic ovaries
Isoechoic ovaries

These patients have an increased risk of ovarian neoplasms occurring in from 5 to 17 %. As normal ovaries show multiple small follicles, a pattern which is present in up to 30 % of polycystic ovary syndrome cases, an apparently normal ultrasound scan does not exclude the diagnosis.

6.7 BILATERAL OVARIAN ENLARGEMENT

Polycystic ovary syndrome (Stein–Leventhal)
Hypothyroidism
McCune Albright syndrome
Ovarian tumours – primary and secondary
Haemorrhage
Cystic disease

6.7.1 Ovarian tumours

Ovarian tumours are uncommon in children and are rare under the age of five years. Those which occur in children (1–2 % of ovarian tumours) are usually benign. The commonest ovarian tumour in childhood is teratoma which is usually benign in young children but 15 % may be malignant in older children. In adult females ovarian tumours are the fourth commonest malignant cause of death with an average five-year survival of 35 %. Benign and malignant tumours cannot be reliably differentiated by ultrasonography but sonography is a sensitive means of detecting ovarian masses. Once detected these masses may be viewed and biopsied at laparoscopy if clinically necessary.

A *Sonographic appearances of ovarian tumours*

Solid mass
Solid mass with cystic component
Echofree mass/cystic mass
Multicystic mass
Echogenic mass with distal shadowing (calcified)

A unilocular ovarian cyst with a simple cyst appearance and a diameter of less than 5 cm is nearly always benign. Multiloculated cysts and cysts with solid components, particularly nodular or papillary components, may be malignant. The presence of ascites in conjunction with a solid or cystic ovarian mass is strongly suspicious of malignancy. However, Meig's syndrome comprises an ovarian tumour, usually a benign fibroma or thecoma, with hydrothorax and ascites. Ovarian tumours may be classified by their epithelial, germ cell or stromal origin. Epithelial tumours are common accounting for 70–80 % of adult and 17 % of paediatric tumours. They are usually benign.

SEROUS CYSTADENOMAS. – The initial appearance is indistinguishable from a simple cyst. They may be bilateral and can undergo malignant change to cyst-adenocarcinoma.

MUCINOUS CYSTADENOMA. – These are usually uni-lateral tumours with a low incidence of malignant change. They may become large and may rupture causing pseudomyxoma peritoneii. Though they may contain echogenic material they cannot usually be differentiated from simple cysts or benign or malignant serous tumours.

Germ cell tumours including dermoids and benign cystic teratomas are also common. They usually present in adolescents and young women but also occur in the elderly. Ten to fifteen per cent are bilateral. Dermoids often contain abnormally differentiated tissue such as fat, teeth and hair and thus their appearance is variable. The majority of dermoids are very echogenic and they may show distal acoustic shadowing. These appearances may be mimicked by bowel loops or calcified uterine fibroids. Fat/fluid levels have been described in cystic tumours. Stromal tumours are uncommon accounting for less than 20 % of ovarian tumours. They include granulosa tumours, fibroma, fibrosarcoma and Sertoli–Leydig tumours. These tumours may secrete hormones and thus may present early. Stromal tumours are usually solid and may be bilateral.

N.B. If a cystic mass is found in the lower abdomen of a female then it is likely to be of ovarian origin whatever its position.

6.7.2 Krukenberg tumours

Krukenberg tumours are metastases within the ovaries though the original description was of ovarian metastatic disease showing signet cell with mucin secretion. Metastases within the ovaries are usually only visible when they cause ovarian enlargement. The commonest appearance is of a pelvic mass usually showing homogenous low level echoes. Fifty per cent of ovarian metastases are from the gastrointestinal tract particularly stomach and colon. Breast tumours and genitourinary malignancy also give rise to ovarian metastases. In children neuroblastoma, lymphoma and leukaemia have also given rise to ovarian metastases.

6.8 OVARIAN TUMOUR ECHOGENICITY

ANECHOIC
  Mucinous cystadenoma
  Serous cystadenoma
  Mucinous cystadenocarcinoma
  Serous cystadenocarcinoma
  Teratoma
MIXED ECHOPATTERN
  Mucinous cystadenoma
  Serous cystadenoma
  Mucinous cystadenocarcinoma
  Serous cystadenocarcinoma
  Adenocarcinoma (without serous or mucin
    secretion)
  Teratoma
  Cystadenofibroma
  Brenner tumour
  Fibrothecoma
  Granulosa cell tumour
  Krukenberg tumour
ECHOGENIC
  Adenocarcinoma (without serous or mucin
    secretion)
  Teratoma
  Brenner tumour
  Fibrothecoma
  Granulosa cell tumour
  Krukenberg tumour

6.8.1 Torsion of the ovary

The majority of cases of ovarian torsion occur secondary to underlying ovarian pathology such as cyst or tumour. The risk of torsion increases with ovarian size particularly with masses over 5 cm in diameter. Sonography may show an ovarian mass due to the underlying pathology or oedema and vascular engorgement. This may be associated with free fluid in the pelvis. Without treatment an old infarcted ovary may calcify.

6.9 PELVIC AND ADNEXAL MASSES

Ovarian cysts e.g.
>   Follicular, corpus luteum, theca lutein,
>   para-ovarian
>   Polycystic ovaries

Ovarian tumours – Primary and secondary

Endometriosis

Ectopic pregnancy

Pelvic inflammatory disease e.g.
>   Hydrosalpinx
>   Tubo-ovarian abscess

Tubal malignancy

Uterine masses including tumours and
  pedunculated fibroids

Pelvic masses arising outside the genital tract:
>   Bowel masses
>   Pelvic malignancy – primary and
>   secondary
>   Pelvic kidney including transplant
>   Haematoma
>   Lymphocoele
>   Bladder masses
>   Sacral tumours
>   Anterior meningocoele
>   Vascular anomalies

6.10 PALPABLE PELVIC MASS NOT SEEN ON ULTRASONOGRAPHY

No true mass present

Mass resolved spontaneously

Mass hidden by bowel loops

Mass mistaken for bowel loops or soft tissues

Mass displaced into the abdomen, the position of a mass may vary depending upon the degree of bladder distension

Large ovarian masses may mimic bladder or ascites

A dermoid or calcified mass giving rise to an echogenic anterior surface with distal shadowing may not give the appearance of a mass

6.11 SONOGRAPHIC PATTERNS OF PELVIC MASSES IN CHILDREN

Cystic adnexal masses:
>   Simple ovarian cyst
>   Cystadenoma
>   Cystadenofibroma
>   Teratoma
>   Hydrosalpinx

Complex adnexal masses:
>   Cyst
>   Teratoma
>   Tubo-ovarian abscess
>   Dysgerminoma
>   Haemorrhagic cyst

Solid adnexal masses:
>   Haemorrhagic cyst
>   Ovarian torsion

      Teratoma
      Dysgerminoma
Uterine/vaginal masses:
      Cystic – hydro/haematometrocolpos
      Complex – Pregnancy
      Solid – Rhabdomyosarcoma
            Hydatidiform mole

6.12 NON-GYNAECOLOGICAL MASSES

Cystic – Abscess
      Enteric duplication
      Ureteral stump
Complex – Sacrococcygeal teratoma
      Abscess
Solid – Haematoma
      Neuroblastoma

6.12.1 Precocious puberty

Eighty per cent of cases of precocious puberty are idiopathic due to early activation of the hypothalamic pituitary axis. Twenty per cent are secondary to encephalitis, hydrocephalus, brain or adrenal tumours. Ultrasonography is valuable as a means of assessing the pelvic organs and exclusion of abdominal and pelvic mass lesions particularly adrenal and ovarian tumours.

(1) Assess the size and configuration of the uterus – child/intermediate/adult configuration
(2) Ovaries – not visible/visible – enlargement symmetrical or asymmetrical

Symmetrical ovarian enlargement with an adult uterine configuration is likely to be due to precocious puberty. Asymmetrical ovarian enlargement is likely to be due to pseudo-precocious puberty. This occurs when female hormone secretion arises from an ovarian or adrenal tumour, ovarian cyst, teratoma, choriocarcinoma or pathology other than the hypothalamic–pituitary axis.

6.13 FLUID IN THE PELVIS

Normal ovulation
Ascites
Pelvic inflammatory disease
Ruptured ovarian cyst
CSF – due to ventriculo-peritoneal shunt
Blood – trauma, post-operation, ectopic
    pregnancy, endometriosis, ruptured ovarian
    cyst e.g. corpus luteum cyst
Post hysterosalpingography
Urine e.g. bladder trauma
Encapsulated collections e.g.
    bowel
    ovarian cyst
    endometriosis
    abscess
    urinoma
    lymphocoele

6.13.1 The uterine tubes

The fallopian tubes cannot usually be differentiated from other pelvic soft tissues unless affected by disease or outlined by ascites within the pelvis. Salpingography may be performed sonographically by injecting sterile saline into the uterus and scanning the abdomen. This allows assessment of tubal patency without the use of ionizing radiation.

A Technique

The pelvis is scanned as a baseline. A vaginal examination is performed and 20 ml of saline is injected into the uterine cavity. Tubal patency is demonstrated by the accumulation of fluid within the pelvis.

6.13.2 Salpingitis

In the acute phase of a first attack of salpingitis pelvic sonography is usually normal and the diagnosis is made clinically. Local spread of infection may give rise to abscess formation which may be demonstrable sonographically but ultrasonic findings are more frequent in recurrent or chronic cases. There may be the non-specific appearance of loss of normal tissue planes with or without the presence of hydro/pyosalpinx which is seen as a fluid collection in or around the uterine tubes. Abscesses vary from very small to large complex masses. Fluid may be seen in the pelvis and the combination of fluid collections with tissue inflammation and thickening may give rise to complex masses.

6.13.3 The pregnant uterus

The possibility of pregnancy should be remembered when scanning the abdomen of any woman of childbearing age. Demonstrating an unexpected pregnancy may prevent further investigation and avoid irradiation of the foetus. Pregnancy may be demonstrated as early as six weeks after the first day of the last menstrual period (four weeks after fertilization).

$5\frac{1}{2}$ weeks – gestational sac visible
6–7 weeks – foetal node visible
7–8 weeks – foetal heart movement becomes visible
8–10 weeks – the placenta is seen as a thickened

part of the gestational ring, it is easily seen by 12
weeks

14 weeks – the kidneys are visible

16 weeks – bladder and stomach are visible. (The
bladder should be visible by 18 weeks)

In early pregnancy the foetus is dated by measuring
the crown–rump length. As the foetus flexes the
accuracy of crown–rump dating decreases and the
cranial biparietal diameter is used. (Crown–rump length
measurement is most accurate for foetal dating in the
6–8 week period. After 12 weeks the biparietal diameter
is used.) Dating a pregnancy sonographically is important as 15–20 % of women cannot accurately remember
their last menstrual period and a further 15 % have
irregular periods.

With a normal pregnancy the human chorionic gonadotrophin (HCG) level correlates with the gestational
sac size up to a diameter of 2.5 cm. A foetal node or
developing foetus should be visible in all normal sacs
of 2.5 cm or greater diameter. Lack of visualization of
a sac or embryo or distortion of the sac strongly
suggests an abnormal pregnancy. A visible sac with a
relatively low HCG level for the sac size occurs in
threatened abortion.

6.13.4 Blighted ovum – anembryonic gestation

A gestational sac may be found without evidence of
foetal parts at a time when they should normally be
visible. Any sac greater than 2.5 cm in diameter without
a foetal node is consistent with a 'blighted ovum' or
anembryonic gestation. The HCG level is positive but
does not show a normal rise with time. The sac may
be distorted or may show internal echoes due to
haemorrhage.

6.13.5 The placenta

The placenta is normally easily seen by 12 weeks of gestation. Its echogenicity is similar to that of the myometrium. By 16 weeks the placenta is the same size as the foetus. The appearance of the placenta may be graded as it matures.

Grade 0 – homogenous pattern bounded by a smooth chorionic plate

Grade 1 – echopattern becomes uneven with echogenic areas

Grade 2 – 'comma' shaped echogenic areas are seen

Grade 3 – increasing placental calcification is seen

Fifty per cent of placentas show calcification by 33 weeks. The mature placenta is usually up to 4 cm thick. Placentas 5 cm or greater in thickness are pathological and may be oedematous.

6.13.6 Abruptio placentae

Abruptio placentae is premature separation of the placenta in the second half of pregnancy. It gives rise to a sonolucent or complex collection beneath the placenta. The haematoma may be mistaken for placental thickening.

6.13.7 Placental infarction

Placental infarction is associated with hypertension and pre-eclampsia. It results in a variable sized sonolucent collection within the placenta.

6.13.8 Intervillous thrombosis

This gives rise to sonolucent space in the placenta.

6.13.9 Chorio-angioma

These vascular malformations or placental haemangiomas occur in 1 % of pregnancies. They cause placental enlargement with an intraplacental mass of variable size which has a complex echopattern.

6.13.10 Placenta previa

Placenta previa is the situation of the placenta over the internal cervical os. As the placenta may migrate cranially during uterine enlargement the diagnosis should only be made late in pregnancy. A posterior placenta previa is unlikely if the distance from the foetal head to the sacrum is 2 cm or less.

6.13.11 Ectopic pregnancy

This serious condition accounts for 10 % of maternal deaths in pregnancy. The diagnosis should be considered in any female of childbearing age who presents with abdominal or pelvic pain and has a history of missed or irregular periods. There has been a threefold increase in incidence of ectopic pregnancy in the USA from 1970 to 1980 and it now occurs in around 14 of every 1000 pregnancies. In 95 % of cases the ectopic foetal implantation occurs in the fallopian tube.

The pregnancy test is a valuable aid to diagnosis. The βHCG pregnancy test becomes positive around the time of the missed period but can be positive as early as one week after conception. If this test is negative then ectopic pregnancy is most unlikely. The βHCG level shows an exponential rise during the first six weeks of pregnancy with the level doubling every 48 h. Failure of this normal rise is a reliable sign of an abnormal pregnancy. Twenty per cent of such cases are due to ectopic pregnancy. Combined intra- and extra-uterine pregnancy is rare occurring in 1 in 16 – 30 000 pregnancies thus demonstration of an intrauterine pregnancy makes ectopic pregnancy unlikely. It should be remembered that endometrial proliferation may mimic a gestational sac and lead to false negative diagnosis. Also the βHCG pregnancy test may be positive before the gestational sac is visible and a patient presenting with pelvic pain at this time may be falsely diagnosed as a case of ectopic pregnancy particularly if there is an alternative pathology such as blood in the pouch of Douglas due to ruptured corpus luteum cyst.

A Sonographic signs of pregnancy

These begin to occur five weeks after the first day of the last menstrual period (i.e. three weeks post fertilization).

A decidual reaction is seen in the endometrium with a small hypoechoic area

A gestational sac becomes visible (clot or decidual cast in the uterus may mimic a sac)

Within the next week the foetal node becomes visible within the sac

SIGNS OF ECTOPIC PREGNANCY –

Absence of an intrauterine pregnancy
(N.B. rarely ectopic and intrauterine pregnancy coincide)

Solid or complex adnexal mass adjacent to an

enlarged but empty uterus. If the ectopic pregnancy is advanced a foetal heart beat may be seen within the mass

Enlarged uterine tube

Decidual reaction/pseudo gestational sac in the uterus

Fluid in the pelvic cul-de-sac (blood)

N.B. loss of foetal viability may cause the pregnancy test to become negative.

ECTOPIC PREGNANCY: DIFFERENTIAL DIAGNOSIS –

Endometriosis

Tubo-ovarian abscess

Appendicitis

Diverticulitis

Torsion of ovarian cyst/neoplasm

Torsion/degeneration of a fibroid

Corpus luteum cyst rupture

N.B. Ectopic pregnancy is a potentially fatal condition. In cases with equivocal sonographic findings laparoscopy may confirm or exclude the diagnosis.

6.13.2 Threatened abortion

Threatened abortion is said to occur when a patient suffers vaginal bleeding during the first trimester. Eighty-five to ninety per cent of these patients proceed to normal delivery. In most cases sonography is unremarkable. The foetus will be visible and will show heart movement. There may be a crescentric lucency around the sac due to the presence of blood. Cases of inevitable abortion have persistent vaginal bleeding. A sac is seen on sonography but the HCG level falls as foetal viability is lost. Cases of missed abortion show an abnormal sac with no evidence of foetal heart movement whilst the sac is absent in complete abortion.

A *Signs of incomplete abortion*

Appearances are variable –

Illdefined fluid collection
Illdefined foetal parts
No visible foetal pole
Sloughing of decidua
Clot in the canal
Dilated cervix

6.14 THE FOETUS

Almost any foetal anomaly which causes major structural changes can be detected by ultrasonography. It should however be remembered that abnormalities may not be evident until organ systems are fully developed. A normal ultrasound scan at 16 weeks cannot therefore exclude major foetal abnormalities. Also, foetal anatomy and physiology change as the foetus develops and an apparent abnormality seen *in utero* may resolve before birth and not be evident in the neonate.

The diagnosis of foetal abnormalities is a complex and exacting task requiring experience and expertise. Misdiagnosis of anomalies can have disastrous consequences both for the foetus and its family and thus obstetric sonography should only be undertaken by those fully trained in this field.

6.14.1 Gestational trophoblastic disease

Hydatidiform mole is an abnormal proliferation of trophoblastic tissue within the uterus. 'Complete' moles consist only of trophoblastic tissue but 'incomplete' moles contain both abnormal trophoblastic tissue and foetal parts. The trophoblastic tissue shows an abnormal chromosomal pattern and is associated with a positive pregnancy test and markedly raised βHCG level. Thirty to fifty per cent of cases also have theca lutein cysts. The uterus is large for dates and contains a mass of trophoblastic tissue which is seen as a mass of mid amplitude echoes consisting of vesicles and areas of haemorrhage. In cases of incomplete mole foetal parts are also visible. A normal foetus, placenta and mole coexist in 1 in 30 000 pregnancies.

6.14.2 Choriocarcinoma

Choriocarcinoma is a rare trophoblastic neoplasm which is usually secondary to an abnormal gestation. The tumour gives rise to an irregular echogenic mass within the uterus surrounded by irregular sonolucent areas due to haemorrhage. The βHCG level is markedly elevated and theca lutein cysts are frequently present. The tumour is aggressive and frequently metastasizes to liver, lung, brain and cervix.

FURTHER READING

Alpern M B *et al*. Sonographic features of paraovarian cysts and their complications. *Am. J. Roent.* (1984) **143**: 157–160.

Athey P A & Malone R S. Sonography of ovarian fibromas/thecomas. *J. Ult. Med.* (1987) **6**: 431–436.

Austin C. Seminars in Ultrasound. **1**(1) March 1980.

Babaknia A *et al*. The Stein Leventhal syndrome and coincidental ovarian tumours. *Obstet. Gynaecol.* (1976) **47**: 223–224.

Baltarowich O H *et al*. The spectrum of sonographic findings in haemorrhagic ovarian cysts. *Am. J. Roent.* (1987) **148**: 901–905.

Berland L L *et al*. Ultrasonic diagnosis of ovarian and adnexal disease. Seminars in Ultrasound. **1**(1) (1980).

Bohlman M E *et al*. Sonographic findings in adenomyosis of the uterus. *Am. J. Roent.* (1987) **148**: 765–766.

Brown T W *et al*. Analysis of ultrasonographic criteria in the evaluation for ectopic pregnancy. *Am. J. Roent.* (1978) **131**: 967–971.

Callen P W *et al*. Intra-uterine contraceptive devices: evaluation by sonography. *Am. J. Roent.* (1980) **135**: 797–800.

Chudleigh P & Pearce J M. *Obstetric Ultrasound*. Churchill Livingstone (1986).

Fleischer A C *et al*. Differential diagnosis of pelvis masses by greyscale sonography. *Am. J. Roent.* (1978) **131**: 469–478.

Frank B *et al*. Sonographic appearances of organised blood within a cyst. 2 case reports. *J. Clin. Ult.* (1975) **3**: 233–234.

Hann L E *et al*. Polycystic ovarian disease: sonographic spectrum. *Am. J. Roent.* (1984) **150**: 531–534.

Helvie M A & Silver T M. Ovarian Torsion: sonographic evaluation. *J. Clin. Ult.* (1989) **17**: (5) 327–332.

Laing F C *et al*. Ultrasonic demonstration of endometrial fluid collections unassociated with pregnancy. *Radiology* (1980) **137**: 471.

Littlewood Teele R *et al*. The radiographic and ultrasonographic evaluation of enteric duplication cysts. *Paed. Rad.* (1980) **10**: 9–14.

McCarthy K A *et al*. Post menopausal fluid collections:

always an indicator of malignancy. *J. Ult. Med.* (1986) **5**: 647–649.

McCarthy S & Taylor K J W. Sonography of vaginal masses. *Am. J. Roent.* (1983) **140**: 1005–1008.

Moyle J W *et al.* Sonography of ovarian tumours. Predictability of tumour type. *Am. J. Roent.* (1983) **141**: 985–991.

Nyberg D A *et al.* Abnormal pregnancy: early diagnosis by US and serum chorionic gonadotrophin levels. *Radiology* (1986) **158**: 393–396.

Pandleska S K *et al.* Splenic torsion presenting as a twisted haemorrhagic ovarian cyst. *Ann. Emerg. Med.* (1985) **14**: 64–66.

Phalke I M. The lost IUCD. *Brit. Med. Ult. Soc. bulletin* **43** (1986): 7.

Quinn S F *et al.* Cystic ovarian teratomas: the sonographic appearance of the dermoid plug. *Radiology* (1985) **14**: 64–66.

Reynolds T *et al.* Sonography of haemorrhagic ovarian cysts. *J. Clin. Ult.* (1986) **14**: 449–453.

Saller J R. Haematometria and haematocolpos ultrasound findings. *Am. J. Roent.* (1979) **132**: 1010.

Sanders R C & James A E (eds). *Principles and Practice of Ultrasonography in Obstetrics and Gynaecology* 3rd Edn. Appleton-Century-Crofts (1985).

Sigel *et al.* Ultrasonography of blood during stasis and coagulation. *Invest. Radiol.* (1981) **16**: 71–76.

Steel W B & Cochrane W J. Eds. *Clinics in Diagnostic Ultrasound 15*. Churchill Livingstone (1984).

Stein I F & Leventhal M L. Amenorrhoea associated with bilateral polycystic ovaries. *Am. J. Obstet. Gynaecol.* (1935) **29**: 181–191.

Taylor K J W. *Atlas of Ultrasonography* (2nd Edn.). Churchill Livingstone (1985).

Thind C R *et al.* The role of ultrasound in the

management of ovarian masses in children. *Clin. Rad.* (1989) **40**: 180–182.

Van Dan P A *et al*. Application of ultrasound in the diagnosis of heterotopic pregnancy – a review of the literature. *J. Clin. Ult.* (1988) **16**: 159–165.

Walsh J W *et al*. Greyscale ultrasound in 204 proved gynaecological masses, accuracy and specific diagnostic criteria. *Radiology* (1979) **130**: 391–397.

Weeks J D *et al*. Greyscale features of haematomas. An ultrasonic spectrum. *Am. J. Roent.* (1978) **131**: 977–980.

Welsh J W *et al*. Greyscale ultrasonography in the diagnosis of endometriosis and adenomyosis. *Am. J. Roent.* (1979) **132**: 87–90.

Wexler J S & McGovern T P. Ultrasonography of female urethral diverticula. *Am. J. Roent.* (1980) **134**: 737–740.

Wicks J D *et al*. Greyscale features of haematomas: an ultrasonic spectrum. *Am. J. Roent.* (1978) **131**: 977–980.

Williams B D & Fisk J D. Sonographic diagnosis of giant urachal cyst in the adult. *Am. J. Roent.* (1981) **136**: 417–418.

Chapter 7

Abdominal Wall, Peritoneum, Retroperitoneum and Miscellaneous Gamuts

7.1 THE SKIN

Sonography of the skin is a valuable means of confirming the presence of subcutaneous cysts or abscesses. Normal appearances of the skin include:

Epidermis – a strongly echogenic layer 1–3 mm thick
Dermis – a homogenous zone less echogenic than epidermis, approximately 3 mm thick
Subcutaneous fat, connective tissue and subcutaneous fat lie deep to the dermis. Though fat attenuates the ultrasound beam the degree of attenuation can differ quite remarkably between different patients. Also, despite this marked attenuation the fat may appear hypoechoic relative to the skin
Skin thickness is increased in acromegaly and is decreased in osteoporosis, Cushing's syndrome and with aging though there is a wide range of appearances

7.1.1. The rectus sheath

The rectus muscles are easily identified in the anterior abdominal wall. They are enclosed in a fibrotic sheath which may trap blood if the abdominal wall is injured thus forming a haematoma. Haematomas are frequently associated with an underlying abnormality which predisposes to haemorrhage such as anticoagulation. Spontaneous haemorrhage may occur in pregnancy, muscular men and old ladies and these cases may present with an acute abdomen. This is usually due to rupture of the inferior epigastric vessels. A haematoma is initially seen as an echofree mass in the anterior abdominal wall. It is one of the few causes of a cystic mass anterior to the bladder though as the blood clots the haematoma may rapidly become echogenic or complex. The haematoma is sharply defined by the limits of the rectus sheath and may have a fusiform configuration.

7.2 DIFFERENTIAL DIAGNOSIS

Abscess
Urachal cyst
Bladder diverticulum
Lymphocoele
Lymphangiomatous cysts
Necrotic tumour
Mesenteric/omental cyst
Enteric duplication
Exophytic hepatic cyst
Pancreatic pseudocyst
Ovarian cyst

7.2.1 The diaphragm

The diaphragm is seen as a curved echogenic sheet. It is traversed by the IVC, oesophagus and aorta at the levels of the 8th, 10th and 12th thoracic vertebral bodies respectively. The diaphragmatic crura may be seen as slightly sonolucent curvilinear structures anterior to and on either side of the abdominal aorta.

A Diaphragmatic movement

Diaphragmatic movement may be assessed with a transverse subxipoid approach with the probe angled upwards allowing both hemidiaphragms to be viewed simultaneously.

7.3 IMPAIRED DIAPHRAGMATIC MOVEMENT

Paralysis
Pulmonary overinflation
Pleural effusion
Empyema
Pulmonary inflammation e.g. embolus or
    infection
Diaphragmatic hernia or eventration
Subphrenic abscess
Abdominal pain
Peritonism
Hepatosplenomegaly
Ascites

7.3.1 Diaphragmatic hernias

A Congenital

Usually posterior Bochdalek hernias. These lie lateral to the spine and occur more frequently on the left than on the right. Anterior Morgagni hernias occur less frequently and are usually smaller.

B Acquired

Traumatic and hiatus hernias. Hiatus hernias may be difficult to see unless outlined by fluid. In cases of doubt examining the abdomen while the patient is drinking may demonstrate the anatomy of the distal oesophagus. When the diaphragm has ruptured bowel loops may be identified passing upwards into the thorax though gas within the bowel loops may obscure the diaphragm. If a pleural effusion is also present then bowel loops can be identified on both sides of the diaphragm more easily.

C Eventration

Eventration is a congenital weakness of the diaphragm. Sonography shows a localized bulge in the diaphragm which contains liver or viscera. Real time sonography may show paradoxical movement of the weak diaphragmatic segment.

7.3.2 Loss of diaphragm echoes

The diaphragm is usually seen as a very well-defined echogenic sheet. Adjacent pleural or ascitic fluid usually enhances diaphragmatic visualization. Loss of continuity of the diaphragm echoes is an uncommon finding but may occur in:

> Rupture/laceration/hernia
> Eventration
> Tumour invasion – directly from lung, pleura or abdomen
> Metastasis
> Primary tumour
> Invasion or organization by adjacent abscess or empyema
> Rupture of hepatic abscess through the diaphragm – rare, consider an amoebic hepatic abscess

Diaphragmatic tumours and cysts are extremely rare,

juxta-diaphragmatic pathology occurs more frequently. Nearly all cases of diaphragmatic tumours, e.g. fibro-sarcoma, occur in adults. They give rise to mass lesions which disrupt diaphragmatic echoes.

Evaluation of right sided diaphragmatic humps and juxta-diaphragmatic masses:

A chest radiograph is usually sufficient for diagnosis but ultrasonography is the next investigation of choice.

Scalloped diaphragm margin – due to hypertrophied muscle bundles, usually seen in deep inspiration or emphysema.

Localized eventration. The diaphragmatic bulge is filled with liver. The area of abnormally weak diaphragm may show paradoxical movement

Fluid collection on either side of the diaphragm

Hernias

7.4 JUXTA-DIAPHRAGMATIC MASSES

Pleuropericardial (spring water) cyst
Pericardial fat pad
Foregut duplication cyst
Aortic aneurysm
Hiatus hernia
Pulmonary cysts, fluid filled bullae, abscess,
  hydatid cyst, sequestration
Subphrenic abscess
Hepatic abscess, neoplasm, cyst, hydatid cyst
Fluid collections e.g. loculated ascites
Hydronephrosis
Herniated kidney

7.4.1 Subphrenic abscess

Appendicitis, perforated peptic ulcer or diverticulum, pelvic inflammatory disease and surgery are the commonest causes of intraperitoneal abscesses. The abscess usually forms in a dependent part of the peritoneal cavity such as the subphrenic and subhepatic spaces and pelvis. In the upper abdomen abscesses occur more frequently in the right subphrenic space than the left. They are seen as fluid collections or complex masses above the liver or spleen closely following the superior contours of these organs. Abscesses may contain debris or even gas giving an echogenic appearance. At times it may be impossible to reliably differentiate a subphrenic abscess from a hepatic abscess. Right sided subphrenic collections may be divided into anterior and posterior collections by the right triangular ligament but these spaces are continuous laterally.

7.5 GIANT CYSTIC MASSES IN CHILDREN

Right upper quadrant
      Hydronephrosis
      Gallbladder hydrops
      Cystic hepatic neoplasm
      Enteric duplication
      Polycystic liver
Left upper quadrant
      Epidermoid cysts of the spleen
      Hydronephrosis
      Enteric duplication
Mid abdomen/epigastrium
      Mesenteric cyst
      Enteric duplication
      Pancreatic pseudocyst
Lower abdomen/pelvis
      Urachal cyst
      Mesenteric cyst
      Enteric duplication
      Serous/mucinous cystadenoma of ovary

7.6 UPPER ABDOMINAL MASSES IN CHILDREN

Echogenic
      Wilms tumour
      Infantile polycystic renal disease
      Neuroblastoma
      Hepatoblastoma
      Hepatoma
Echogenic with hypoechoic areas
      Wilms tumour
      Mesoblastic nephroma
      Hepatoblastoma
      Neuroblastoma
Hypoechoic with echogenic areas
    Hepatic hamartoma
    Hepatic adenoma
    Lymphoma
    Cystic neuroblastoma
    Cavernous haemangioblastoma
    Teratoma
    Metastases e.g. testicular embryonal cell
      carcinoma
    Haematoma
    Anechoic
      Abscess
      Choledochal cyst
      Benign cystic hepatoblastoma
      Lymphoma
      Urinoma
      Haematoma

7.7　NEONATAL ABDOMINAL MASSES

Renal (55 %)
    Hydronephrosis (25 %) e.g. urethral
       valves, PUJ obstruction, ureterocoele
    Multicystic kidney (15 %)
    Infantile polycystic disease
    Renal vein thrombosis
    Renal ectopia
    Wilms tumour
    Mesoblastic nephroma
Genital (15 %)
    Ovarian cyst
    Hydro/haemometrocolpos
Gastrointestinal
    Bowel duplication
    Mesenteric cyst
Retroperitoneal (non-renal)
    Adrenal haemorrhage
    Neuroblastoma
    Teratoma
Hepato/spleno/biliary
    Hepatoblastoma
    Hepatic cyst
    Splenic haematoma
    Choledochal cyst

7.8 SONOGRAPHIC APPEARANCES OF PELVIC MASSES IN FEMALE CHILDREN

Cystic adnexal masses
     Ovarian cyst
     Teratoma
     Cystadenoma
     Cystadenofibroma
     Hydrosalpinx
Complex adnexal masses
     Ovarian cyst
     Teratoma
     Tubo-ovarian abscess
     Haemorrhagic cyst
     Dysgerminoma
Solid adnexal mass
     Haemorrhagic cyst
     Ovarian torsion
     Teratoma
     Dysgerminoma
Uterine/vagina
     Pregnancy
     Hydrometrocolpos
     Hydatidiform mole
     Rhabdomyosarcoma
Non-gynaecological masses
     Abscess
     Bowel duplication
     Ureteral stump
     Sacrococcygeal teratoma
     Haematoma
     Neuroblastoma
     Distended bowel e.g. Hirschsprung's
     Distended bladder
     Extramedullary haemopoiesis

Sacrococcygeal chordoma
Ectopic kidney
Meconium pseudocyst
Cloacal dysgenesis

7.9 COMPLEX CYSTIC MASSES IN THE LOWER ABDOMEN IN ADULTS

(A complex cystic mass may have either a cystic appearance with internal septae or debris or both solid and cystic elements)

Ovarian masses e.g. Simple cyst, Cystadenoma/cystadenocarcinoma, Haemorrhagic cyst, Polycystic ovary

Infection e.g. pyogenic abscess, tuberculous psoas abscess, hydatid cyst

Haematoma in bowel wall, mesentery, rectus sheath or retroperitoneum

Renal masses particularly in an ectopic or ptotic kidney e.g. hydronephrosis, polycystic kidney, necrotic neoplasm, dilated tortuous ureter, ureterocoele

Bowel. Adjacent loops of fluid filled small bowel, inflammatory bowel mass, duplication cyst

Benign mesenteric cysts, cystic mesenteric tumour

Benign retroperitoneal cysts, cystic retroperitoneal tumour

Cystic lymphangioma of mesentery or retroperitoneum

Chylous cyst

Post-traumatic uriniferous pseudocyst

Lymphocoele

Endometriosis

Hydro/pyosalpinx
Haematometra/pyometrium
Necrotic endometrial carcinoma or
  leiomyosarcoma
Necrotic retroperitoneal tumour e.g. sarcoma
Cystic teratoma or dermoid
Ectopic pregnancy
Incarcerated Spigelian hernia
Urachal cyst
Ventriculo-peritoneal pseudocyst
Any large upper abdominal cyst extending
  into the lower abdomen

7.9.1 The peritoneum

The peritoneum is a thin serous membrane lining the abdominal cavity. It has parietal and visceral layers, the latter being reflected over the abdominal viscera. The two layers are separated by a thin layer of serous fluid which acts as a lubricant. Several intra-abdominal organs are invaginated by visceral peritoneum to such an extent that they are almost completely covered by peritoneum and carry double layers of peritoneum with them as mesenteries and ligaments.

7.9.2 The falciform ligament

This is a double layer of peritoneum which forms anteriorly near the midline between the umbilicus and oesophagus. It passes backwards and splits to enclose the liver. Superiorly peritoneal layers form the triangular and coronary ligaments which enclose the bare area of the liver. The layers of peritoneum investing the liver unite on its visceral surface to form the lesser omentum which passes from the liver to the oesophagus, stomach and first part of the duodenum. The free edge of the lesser omentum between the porta hepatis and the duodenum contains the portal vein with the hepatic artery and common bile duct lying antero-medial and antero-lateral respectively. The layers of the lesser omentum split to enclose the stomach and then re-unite to form the greater omentum and gastrosplenic and lieno-renal ligaments.

7.9.3 Ascites

Ascitic fluid is seen as echofree fluid between the bowel loops. With small volumes the location of the fluid is very dependent upon the patient's position. In these cases the fluid tends to gravitate into the pelvis or paracolic gutters. Traces of fluid may frequently be seen in the flanks, around the liver and between the liver and right kidney. With larger volumes of fluid the bowel loops float rising to the centre of the abdomen which is obscured by bowel gas. (Pseudomyxoma peritoneii may give a similar appearance but may encase the bowels or lie anterior to the bowels which do not float in the fluid to the same extent as occurs with ascites.)

The presence of debris within ascites is suggestive of tuberculosis or haemoperitoneum. Septations may occur in chronic pyogenic peritonitis, pseudomyxoma peritoneii or peritoneal – atrial shunt whilst mottled or thick walled bowel loops suggest malignancy or bowel inflammation.

7.9.4 Differential diagnosis

Loculated ascites may be mimicked by:
    Gallbladder hydrops
    Abscess

Blood – post-operation, trauma, bleeding diathesis, leaking aneurysm
Chylous ascites
Dialysis fluid
Cerebrospinal fluid (from VP shunt)
Urine

A Ascites – aetiology

Transudates e.g. cardiac failure, hypoalbuminaemia, hypoproteinaemia, IVC obstruction, portal hypertension and cirrhosis.

Exudates, peritoneal inflammation, peritoneal malignancy.

Urine, due to intraperitoneal rupture of the urinary tract.

Chylous ascites. Secondary to congenital or acquired lymphatic obstruction though slight chylous ascites is not uncommon in the newborn. Acquired chylous ascites may occur secondary to lymphatic obstruction which may complicate tumours, trauma, radiotherapy, filariasis.

Blood, due to trauma, penetrating injury, hepatic or splenic laceration. Also due to spontaneous rupture of an intra-abdominal structure such as an ovarian cyst.

CSF. Loculation of CSF around a shunt usually occurs in the presence of peritoneal adhesions which reduce the peritoneal surface available for resorption. The ventriculo-peritoneal shunt tubing may be identified within the collection.

Meconium peritonitis. Meconium peritonitis is a chemical peritonitis which occurs when meconium leaks from the bowel into the peritoneum in the foetus. Inflammation may block the bowel leak thus evidence of previous meconium peritonitis may be the only sign of an earlier bowel abnormality. In other cases meconium peritonitis is secondary to underlying disease such as bowel atresia or stenosis which will also be evident. The peritoneal meconium calcifies giving rise to curvilinear and irregular areas of calcification. *In utero* there may be evidence of polyhydramnios, ascites and bowel abnormalities. Cases of meconium peritonitis giving rise to a 'snow storm' appearance have been recorded due to the presence of multiple fine calcified particles floating in the ascitic fluid. These abnormalities may persist after birth giving rise to abdominal cysts and calcifications.

7.9.5 Peritoneal metastases

Peritoneal metastases may arise from any primary site but particularly gastrointestinal tract, kidney, pancreas, breast and the pelvic organs. When visible the peritoneum is seen as the peritoneal line which comprises both peritoneum and deep abdominal fascia. This is most clearly demonstrated by scanning with a high frequency probe. When extraperitoneal fat is abundant the peritoneum and fascia are seen as two separate lines. Peritoneal metastases may present as:

Ascites
Peritoneal masses projecting as polypoid masses into the ascitic fluid. These may be nodular, sheet like or irregular (Fig. 15). Metastases may grow and become adherent to adjacent organs
Adhesions between bowel loops
Masses between bowel loops

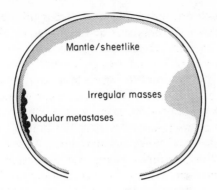

Fig. 15. Sonographic appearances of peritoneal metastases. When small, peritoneal metastases are difficult to identify and are easily missed. The presence of ascites makes it easier to visualize small metastatic deposits which may show the above patterns.

   Bowel fixation – firm pressure with the transducer
      fails to displace bowel loops
   Extensive adhesions may obliterate part of the
      peritoneal cavity
   The peritoneal line may be broken by metastatic
      invasion

N.B. Even extensive peritoneal metastatic disease may not be evident sonographically if there is little or no ascites present and serosal metastases are obscured by gas within the bowel loops.

A Differential diagnosis
Peritoneal mesothelioma – gives rise to sheet-like nodular or irregular mass lesions. Most cases are associated with ascites.

Appendices epiploicae of the large bowel may be visible in the presence of ascites. These are seen at regular intervals along the large bowel.

7.9.6 The omental bursa (lesser sac)

The lesser sac is a peritoneal recess lying behind the stomach. It communicates with the peritoneal cavity via the foramen of Winslow and is bounded anteriorly by the liver, lesser omentum, stomach and greater omentum from above downwards. The posterior abdominal wall, duodenum IVC and pancreas lie posteriorly. The lesser sac may be visualized when distended by pathological fluid collections such as loculated ascites or pancreatic pseudocyst.

7.9.7 The retroperitoneum

The retroperitoneum comprises the organs and fascial spaces lying posterior to the peritoneal cavity and anterior to the muscles of the posterior abdominal wall. Retroperitoneal structures include the major vessels and adjacent lymphatics, kidneys, adrenal glands, pancreas and psoas muscles. Disease of any of these organs may affect the retroperitoneum and disease from other areas may affect the retroperitoneum either by direct spread or indirectly via the blood vessels or lymphatics.

7.9.8 Anechoic retroperitoneal masses

Retroperitoneal varices – serpiginous anechoic structures

Sarcoma – most appear as anechoic or hypoechoic masses

Other tumour masses, in particular lymphoma

deposits

Lymphadenopathy, metastatic or inflammatory

Haematoma – anechoic/hypoechoic/septate/complex (appearance depends upon the age of the haematoma)

Abscess – may be indistinguishable from haematoma

Retroperitoneal fibrosis – this may give rise to a retroperitoneal mantle of tissue of low or moderate echogenicity around the major vessels which has a well defined anterior margin but a poorly defined posterior margin. It is not easily separated from adjacent structures and tends to envelope the IVC and aorta without causing displacement

Aortic aneurysm (lymph nodes around the aorta may mimic an aneurysm)

Retroperitoneal lymphangiomatosis and lymphangiomyomatosis – cystic structures around the aorta and IVC, may appear septate

7.9.9 The aorta

The aorta can usually be visualized throughout most of its abdominal course by an anterior approach in slim patients but in obese patients a left posterior oblique approach may be required scanning through the left kidney. Ultrasonography is now the initial investigation of choice in patients with pulsatile abdominal masses. It allows:

Accurate measurement of the aneurysm diameter

It will show the configuration of the aneurysm

It will show clot within the aneurysm which may make an aneurysm look artificially small on angiography

The aneurysm wall thickness may be measured, the

wall is thicker in inflammatory/infective aneurysms than in atheromatous aneurysms

Dissection may be demonstrated

Haematoma around a leaking aneurysm may be
shown

A normal aorta with an overlying mass can be
differentiated from an aneurysm. (Echolucent
lymphnodes in cases of lymphoma may mimic an
aneurysm)

A   Normal maximum diameter

At the diaphragm: 2.5 cm
Mid abdomen: 2.0 cm
At the bifurcation: 1.8 cm
Iliac arteries: 1.0 cm

The aorta should always be examined in both transverse and longitudinal sections as oblique sections
exaggerate the aortic dimensions. Imaging in multiple
planes is particularly important if the aorta is tortuous.
An aortic aneurysm is seen as a dilatation of the aorta.
The aneurysm may contain a variable amount of clot
which is relatively hypoechoic but is more echogenic
than the remaining aortic lumen which is anechoic.
The majority of aortic aneurysms are fusiform though
they may be saccular or eccentric. They frequently
extend into the iliac arteries though proximally they
usually arise below the level of the renal arteries.
Turbulent flow may be seen within an aneurysm and
blood or clot may be seen outside the aortic lumen in
cases of leaking or false aneurysms.

B Aortic aneurysms diameter < 6 cm

1 year survival 75 %
5 year survival 47.8 %

C Aortic aneurysms diameter > 6 cm

1 year survival 50 %
2 year survival 25 %
5 year survival 6 %

(Overall risk of rupture 43 % – other deaths from related cardiovascular episodes etc.)

D Aortic aneurysm, differential diagnosis

Anechoic para-aortic nodes
Para-aortic/para-vertebral haematoma
Oblique sections through a tortuous aorta
Fluid filled small bowel loops over the anterior aortic
  wall
Loculated ascites in the mid abdomen

7.9.10 The inferior vena cava

The inferior vena cava (IVC) forms by the union of the common iliac veins at the level of the 5th lumbar vertebral body. It ascends on the right side of the aorta to the level of the second lumbar vertebral body at which point it is directed slightly forwards through the liver. The right renal artery can usually be seen passing behind the IVC just before it enters the liver and the IVC usually shows posterior indentation at this point. IVC distension varies with respiration, position and the cardiac cycle. Distension occurs in cases of right heart failure, fluid overload and other causes of raised central venous pressure. As the IVC distends calibre changes normally seen with respiration become less marked and eventually cease.

7.9.11   Intraluminal IVC mass (Intraluminal echoes in a distended IVC)

Tumour thrombi – may enter the IVC via renal, adrenal, hepatic veins etc. Commonest cause is extension of renal tumour. Also hepatic, adrenal and retroperitoneal tumours both benign and malignant, e.g. carcinomas, sarcoma, teratoma, lymphoma.

Non-tumour thrombi e.g. extension of deep venous thrombosis

Primary IVC tumour e.g. leiomyosarcoma

Foreign body e.g. IVC filter

7.10 MASSES THAT ELEVATE THE IVC

The cranial section of the IVC is nearly always
  visible though the caudal part is frequently
  obscured by bowel loops. It may be
  elevated by retroperitoneal masses:
Right adrenal tumour
Neurogenic tumours
Hepatic masses in the posterior aspect of the
  caudate and right lobes
Right renal artery aneurysm
Renal mass
Lymphadenopathy
Dilated retrocaval ureter (non-dilated
  retrocaval ureter does not usually elevate
  the IVC)
Retroperitoneal tumour
Lumbar spine disease
Tortuous aorta
Haematoma
Abscess
Retroperitoneal fibrosis

7.12 INFERIOR VENA CAVA OBSTRUCTION

IVC shows loss of kinetics – loss of calibre
change with respiration
Solid pattern in the lumen
Decreased or absent Doppler signal
Abnormal Doppler signal/turbulent flow
Colateral channels
Differential diagnosis:
Extrinsic compression e.g. nodes or
retroperitoneal masses
Retroperitoneal fibrosis

7.12.1 Abdominal lymphatics

The lymphatics of the anterior and lateral abdominal
walls drain to the axillary, anterior mediastinal and
superficial inguinal lymph nodes. The lymphatics of
the abdominal viscera drain to the lymph nodes around
the aorta. The lymph nodes around the aorta lie around
the origins of the coelic axis, superior and inferior
mesenteric arteries anteriorly and around the paired
lateral aortic branches. Any or all the pre-aortic and
para-aortic lymph nodes may be enlarged by tumour
infiltration or inflammatory disease. Early lymphadenopathy is most easily identified when the pre-aortic
nodes are involved as masses around the origins of
the anterior aortic branches distort and elevate these
vessels. Enlarged lymph nodes are usually hypoechoic
in relation to adjacent retroperitoneal tissue but they
may be echogenic. Lymphoma in particular gives rise
to large anechoic nodes. When enlarged pre- and para-
aortic nodes are identified the bowel mesentery should
be reviewed for evidence of lymphadenopathy and the
abdominal organs should be examined for evidence of

an occult primary tumour. If an occult primary tumour is suspected then examination of the testes and thyroid should also be undertaken.

FURTHER READING

Alonso de Santos L & Goldstein H M. Ultrasonography in tumours arising from the spine and bony pelvis. *Am. J. Roent.* (1977) **129**: 1061–1064.

Bailey R V *et al*. Leiomyosarcoma of the inferior vena cava: a report of a case and review of the literature. *Ann. Surg.* (1976) **184**: 169–173.

Bresenihan E R & Keates P G. Ultrasound of dissection of the abdominal aorta. *Clin. Rad.* (1980) **3**: 105–108.

Bruyninck C M A & Derkson O S. Leiomyosarcoma of the IVC: a case report and review of the literature. *J. Vasc. Surg.* (1986) **3**: 652–656.

Callen P W *et al*. Ascitic fluid in the anterior perivesical fossa: misleading appearance on CT scans. *Am. J. Roent.* (1978) **130**: 1176–1177.

Campbell J A. The diaphragm in roentgenology of the chest. *Rad. Clin. North Am.* (1963) 395–410.

Campbell W E & Weinstein B J. Sonographic appearances of pelvic extramedullary haematopoiesis. *J. Ult. Med.* (1986) **5**: 103–104.

Creed L *et al*. Potential pitfalls in CT and sonographic evaluation of suspected lymphoma. *Am. J. Roent.* (1982) **139**: 606–607.

Derchi L E *et al*. Appendices epiploicae of the large bowel: sonographic appearances and differentiation from peritoneal seeding. *J. Ult. Med.* (1988) **7**: 11–14.

Didier D *et al*. Tumour thrombus of the IVC secondary to malignant abdominal neoplasm: ultrasound and CT evaluation. *Radiology* (1987) **162**: 83–89.

Didier D *et al*. Hepatic alveolar echinococcus: correlative ultrasound and CT study. *Radiology* (1985) **154**: 179–186.

Edell S L & Gefter W B. Ultrasonic differentiation of types of ascitic fluid. *Am. J. Roent.* (1979) **133**: 111–114.

Fagan C J *et al*. Retroperitoneal fibrosis: ultrasound and CT features. *Am. J. Roent.* (1979) **133**: 239–243.

Feinstein K A & Fernboch S K. Septated urinomas in the neonate. *Am. J. Roent.* (1987) **149**: 997–1000.

Hardin W J & Hardy J O. Mesenteric cysts. *Am. J. Surg.* (1970) **119**: 640.

Johnson A R *et al*. Tailgut cyst: diagnosis with CT and sonography. *Am. J. Roent.* (1986) **147**: 1309–1311.

Kangarloo H *et al*. Ultrasonic evaluation of juxtadiaphragmatic masses in children. *Radiology* (1977) **125**: 785–787.

Khan A N & Gould D A. The primary role of ultrasound in evaluating right sided diaphragmatic humps and juxtadiaphragmatic masses. *Clin. Rad.* (1984) **35**: 413–418.

Khan A N & Bisset R A L. A complex cystic abdominal mass: an unusual presentation of Crohn's disease in an anticoagulated patient. *J. Clin. Ult.* (1988) **16**: 271–274.

Kordon B & Payne S D. Fat necrosis simulating a primary tumour of the mesentery – sonographic diagnosis. *J. Ult. Med.* (1988) **7**: 345–347.

Kurtz A B *et al*. Ultrasound diagnoses of masses elevating the IVC. *Am. J. Roent.* (1979) **132**: 401–406.

Kutcher R *et al*. Renal angiomyolipoma with sonographic demonstration of extension into the IVC. *Radiology* (1982) **143**: 755–756.

Lee T G & Henderson S C. Ultrasonic aortography:

unexpected findings. *Am. J. Roent.* (1977) **128**: 273–276.

Li *et al*. Pseudoperisplenic 'fluid collections': A clue to normal liver and spleen echogenic texture. *J. Ult. Med.* (1986) **5**: 397–400.

Mariona F *et al*. Sonographic detection of foetal extra-thoracic pulmonary sequestration. *J. Ult. Med.* (1986) **5**: 283–285.

Murphy N B. Abdominal aortic ultrasonography – a valuable diagnostic technique. *J. Irish Med. Assoc.* (1977) **70**: 231–233.

Perry M *et al*. Causes of abnormal right diaphragmatic position diagnosed by ultrasound. *J. Clin. Ult.* (1983) **11**: 269–275.

Pussel S J & Cosgrove D O. Ultrasound features of tumour thrombus in the IVC in retroperitoneal tumours. *Brit. J. Rad.* (1981) **5**: 866–869.

Rao I C G & Woodlief R M. Greyscale ultrasonic demonstration of rupture right hemidiaphragm. *Brit. J. Rad.* (1980) **53**: 812–814.

Raymond H W & Zweiber W J. *Seminars in Ultrasound.* (1980) Vol 1 No 3.

Schwartz S I *et al*. Tumours of the mesentery. In *Principles of Surgery* (McGraw Hill 1974), p. 1334.

Schwerk W B *et al*. Venous renal tumour extension: a prospective ultrasound evaluation. *Radiology* (1985) **156**: 491–495.

Spring D B *et al*. The sonographic appearance of fluid in the prevesical space. *Radiology* (1983) **147**: 205–206.

Spring D B *et al*. Ultrasonic evaluation of lymphocoele formation after staging lymphadenectomy for prostatic carcinoma. *Radiology* (1981) **141**: 479–483.

Subramanyah B R *et al*. Hepatocellular carcinoma with

venous invasion: sonographic-angiographic correlation. *Radiology* (1984) **150**: 793–796.

Walsh J *et al*. Greyscale ultrasonography in retroperitoneal lymphangiomatosis. *Am. J. Roent.* (1977) **129**: 1101–1102.

Wheeler W E *et al*. Angiography and ultrasonography: a comparative study of abdominal aortic aneurysms. *Am. J. Roent.* (1976) **126**: 95–100.

Wicks J D *et al*. Giant cystic abdominal masses in children and adolescents: ultrasonic differential diagnosis. *Am. J. Roent.* (1978) **130**: 853–857.

Worthen N J & Worthen W F. Disruption of diaphragmatic echoes: a sonographic sign of diaphragmatic disease. *J. Clin. Ult.* (1982) **10**: 43–45.

Wu A & Siegel M J. Sonography of pelvic masses in children: diagnostic predictability. *Am. J. Roent.* (1987) **149**: 997–1000.

Yeh H C. Ultrasonography of peritoneal tumours. *Radiology* (1979) **133**: 419–422.

Yeh H C & Chahinien A P. Ultrasonography and computed tomography of peritoneal mesothelioma. *Radiology* (1980) **135**: 705–712.

Index